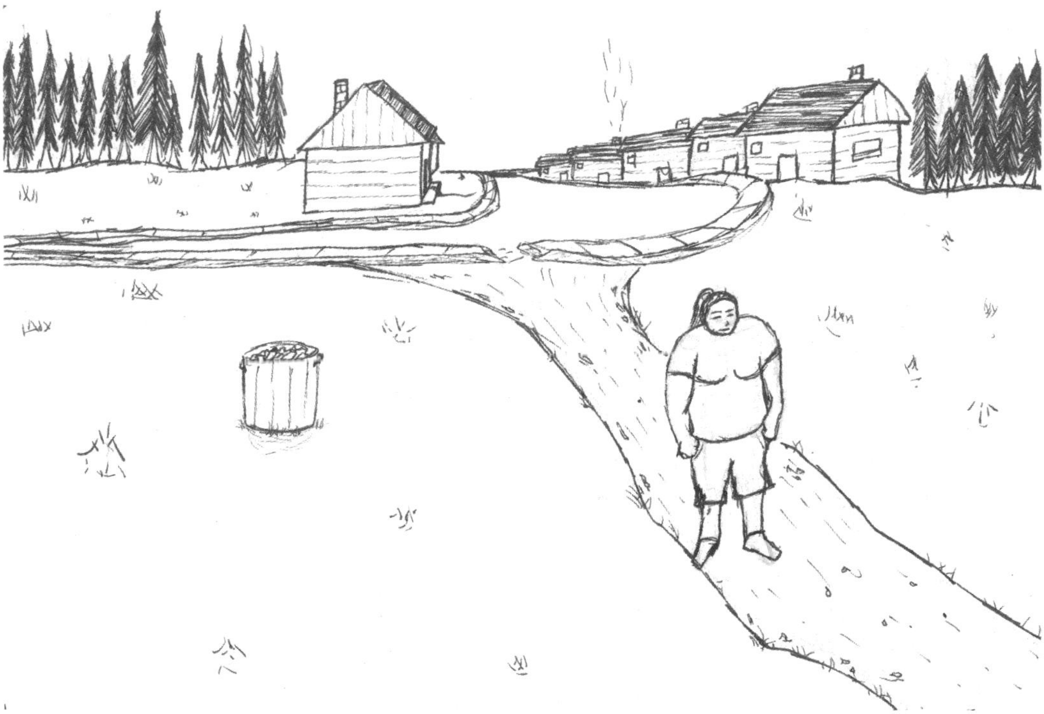

# ᒉᓂᕗᕐ ᑫ·ᓛᕆᔮ ᓗᐯᔅ ᐅᑎᐹᒋᒧ·ᐃᓐ ·ᐚ·ᓵᓂᐲᐦᒡ ᐅᐦᒌᐤ

# ᒉᓂᕗᕐ ᑲ·ᓛᕆᔮ ·ᓛᐯᔅ ᐅᑎᐹᒋᒧ·ᐃᓐ, ·ᐚᔅ·ᐋᓂᐲᐅᐄᓅ

## L’histoire de Jennifer Gloria Lowpez de Waswanipi

## The Story of Jennifer Gloria Lowpez of Waswanipi


Told by Jennifer Gloria Lowpez
Written by Ruth DyckFehderau
Translated into Northern East Cree by Luci Bobbish-Salt
Translated into Southern East Cree by Louise Blacksmith
Translated into French by Valérie Duro



ᒋᔦᐲᒪᑎᓰᐅᓐ ᐊᓈᓈᑭᒋᐦᒑᑭᓅᒃ
CONSEIL CRI DE LA SANTÉ ET DES SERVICES SOCIAUX DE LA BAIE JAMES
CREE BOARD OF HEALTH AND SOCIAL SERVICES OF JAMES BAY

Funding for this publication was provided in part by Health Canada. The opinions expressed in this publication are those of the storyteller and do not necessarily reflect the official views of Health Canada or of the Cree Board of Health and Social Services of James Bay.

Some names and details in this book have been changed for the purpose of protecting identities. Any similarities between these changed names or details and real persons, living or dead, is not intended.

First printing, 2020. Printed and bound in Canada by Houghton Boston Printers, Saskatoon, Saskatchewan. Distributed by Wilfrid Laurier University Press / wlupress.wlu.ca

Set in Verdana font, chosen for its readability. Printed on paper that is Forest Stewardship Council-certified with post-consumer recycled fibres, and that is acid- and chlorine-free.

Cover design by Nicole Ritzer, based on an original design by Cameron Mosimann. Photograph of Mistissini burnt forest (reversed) taken by David DyckFehderau. Title page illustration by Jewyll Brien of Mikw Chiyâm Arts Concentration Program, Voyageur Memorial High School, Mistissini, QC.


Published by Cree Board of Health and Social Services of James Bay
Contact: Paul Linton, 168 Main St, Mistissini, QC, Canada, G0W 1C0 / (418) 923-3355
creehealth.org / sweetbloods.org

Library and Archives Canada Cataloguing in Publication

Title: Chenivir kilwaariyaa lupes utipaachimuwin waaswaanipiihch uhchiiu = Chenivir kalwaariyaa lwaapes utipaachimuwin, waaswaanipiiuiinuu = L'histoire de Jennifer Gloria Lowpez de Waswanipi = The story of Jennifer Gloria Lowpez of Waswanipi / story by Jennifer Gloria Lowpez ; translator Northern East Cree, Luci Bobbish-Salt ; translator Southern East Cree, Louise Blacksmith ; translator French Valérie Duro ; writer, Ruth DyckFehderau.

Other titles: Chenivir kalwaariyaa lwaapes utipaachimuwin, waaswaanipiiuiinuu | Histoire de Jennifer Gloria Lowpez de Waswanipi | Story of Jennifer Gloria Lowpez of Waswanipi

Names: DyckFehderau, Ruth, author. | DyckFehderau, Ruth, 1967-. Story of Jennifer Gloria Lowpez of Waswanipi. | DyckFehderau, Ruth, 1967- Story of Jennifer Gloria Lowpez of Waswanipi. Cree. | DyckFehderau, Ruth, 1967- Story of Jennifer Gloria Lowpez of Waswanipi. French. | Cree Board of Health and Social Services of James Bay, issuing body.

Description: Cree title romanized. | "This is a four-language translation of a single story from The Sweet Bloods of Eeyou Istchee: Stories of Diabetes and the James Bay Cree. (Sweet Bloods contains 26 stories.)" | Text in Northern East Cree, Southern East Cree, French, and English.

Identifiers: Canadiana 2020040234XE | ISBN 9781989796030 (softcover)

Subjects: LCSH: Lowpez, Jennifer Gloria—Health. | LCSH: Addicts—Waswanipi (First Nation)—Biography. | LCSH: Diabetics—Waswanipi (First Nation)—Biography. | LCGFT: Biographies.

Classification: LCC HV5805.L69 D93 2020 | DDC 362.29092—dc23

Catalogage avant publication de Bibliothèque et Archives Canada
Titre: Chenivir kilwaariyaa lupes utipaachimuwin waaswaanipiihch uhchiiu = Chenivir kalwaariyaa lwaapes utipaachimuwin, waaswaanipiiuiinuu = L'histoire de Jennifer Gloria Lowpez de Waswanipi = The story of Jennifer Gloria Lowpez of Waswanipi / story by Jennifer Gloria Lowpez ; translator Northern East Cree, Luci Bobbish-Salt ; translator Southern East Cree, Louise Blacksmith ; translator French Valérie Duro ; writer, Ruth DyckFehderau.
Autres titres: Chenivir kalwaariyaa lwaapes utipaachimuwin, waaswaanipiiuiinuu | Histoire de Jennifer Gloria Lowpez de Waswanipi | Story of Jennifer Gloria Lowpez of Waswanipi
Noms: DyckFehderau, Ruth, 1967- auteur. | DyckFehderau, Ruth, 1967- Story of Jennifer Gloria Lowpez of Waswanipi. | DyckFehderau, Ruth, 1967- Story of Jennifer Gloria Lowpez of Waswanipi. Cree. | DyckFehderau, Ruth, 1967- Story of Jennifer Gloria Lowpez of Waswanipi. Français. | Conseil Cri de la santé et des services sociaux de la Baie-James, organisme de publication.
Description: Titre cri romanisé. | Publiée antérieurement dans : The Sweet Bloods of Eeyou Istchee: Stories of Diabetes and the James Bay Cree. | Texte en cri de l'Est du nord, en cri de l'Est du sud, en français et en anglais.
Identifiants: Canadiana 2020040234XF | ISBN 9781989796030 (couverture souple)
Vedettes-matière: RVM: Lowpez, Jennifer Gloria—Santé. | RVM: Dépendants—Waswanipi (Première nation)—Biographies. | RVM: Diabétiques—Waswanipi (Première nation)—Biographies. | RVMGF: Biographies.
Classification: LCC HV5805.L69 D93 2020 | CDD 362.29092—dc23

ᐧᐃᔮᔥ 2007 ᑳ ᐄᒋᔥᑖᔨᒡ ᐋᐦ ᐱᐳᓂᔨᒡ, ᓂᒧᐃ ᓈᔥᒡ ᐅᐦᒋ ᒥᔦᐱᔨᔨᐤ ᓛᐧᑳᔨᐤ ᒉᓂᕕᕐ ᑭᐧᒑᓇᔮ ᒍᐯᔅ ᐧᐄᒋᐧᐋᐦᑊᒡ᙮ ᐹᔨᐧᑳᐤ ᐋᐦ ᑎᐱᔅᑳᔨᒡ ᑳ ᐅᑎᓂᐦᒃ ᓂᑐᐦᑯᔨᓐᐦ, ᒥᐦᒑᑐ ᓂᑐᐦᑯᔨᓐᐦ, ᐋᑯᐦ ᒥᓂᐦᐧᑳᐅᑭᒥᑯᐦᑊᒡ ᑳ ᐄᑐᐦᑖᑦ ᐋᑯᑎᐦ ᑳ ᒥᓂᐦᐧᑳᑦ ᑳᐲᔥᒑᐅᐲᔑᔨᒡ ᑮᔮᐦ ᔔᒥᓈᐳᔨᐤ ᑮᔮᐦ ᓴᒥᔨᐤ ᑮᔮᐦ ᐧᕚᑎᑳ᙮ ᑳ ᐅᑎᓂᐦᒃ ᐱᐧᔮᐱᔅᑯᔫᑭᓂᔨᐤ ᐋᐦ ᒌᐦ ᔒᑯᔥᑎᑭᓂᐧᐃᐧᐃᔨᒡ, ᑳ ᐲᐦᑯᐦᑖᑦ, ᑮᔮᐦ ᑳ ᒫᒋᔓᑯᑦ ᐅᒥᐦᐧᑳᔫᐲᐦᑊᒡ᙮ ᑳ ᐱᐦᒋᔑᐦᒃ ᑮᔮᐦ ᑳ ᓂᑭᑎᑯᑦ ᐅᑎᐦᒑᐦᑯᐦ ᑮᔮᐦ ᑳᐦ ᓂᑭᑎᐦᒃ ᐊᓂᔮ ᐅᔦ ᒥᔥᑏᐦ ᐋᐦ ᓂᑭᑎᑯᑦ ᐅᒥᐦᑯ ᒫᐧᑳᒡ ᐋᐦ ᐱᒥᔑᐦᒃ ᐊᓂᑎᐦ ᓂᐱᒋᔅᑎᑯᐦᑊᒡ ᓈᔥᒡ ᐋᐦ ᐧᐄᓈᔨᒡ᙮

ᑳ ᐹᐦᑎᐧᐋᑦ ᐊᐧᐋᔨᐤᐦ ᐋᐦ ᐋᔨᒥᐦᐄᑯᑦ ᐅᐦᑑᑳᐦᑊᒡ, “ᐋᑯᑎᐦ ᐅᑎᐦ ᐃᐦᑖᐦ, ᒉᓂᕕᕐ, ᒋᓂᑎᐧᐋᔨᒥᑯᒡ ᐧᐋᔥ ᐊᔥᑎᐧᐋᔑᔒᒥᒡ᙮” ᐋᐦᑖᐧᐋᐧᑳ ᐊᐧᐋᔑᔑᒡ ᑮᔮᐦ ᒫᒃ ᐋᑦ ᐧᐋᑲ ᐃᐦᑖᐧᐋᐧᑳ ᐊᐧᐋᔑᔑᒡ, ᔖᔥ ᐄᔑᓈᑯᓐ ᒑ ᒫᒋᔮᓐ᙮ ᐋᑯᐦ ᔖᔥ ᐅᑎᐦᒋᐱᔨᐤ ᒑ ᒫᒋᔮᓐ᙮

ᐊᓂᑖᐦ ᒫᒃ ᔑᐳᑯᒨ ᓂᑐᐦᑯᔨᓂᑭᒥᑯᐦᑊᒡ ᐋᑯᑖᐦ ᑳᐦ ᐅᐦᒋ ᐧᐃᓂᔥᑳᑦ ᒉᓂᕕᕐ᙮ ᐊᓂᔮᐦ ᐊᐧᐋᔨᐤᐦ, ᐧᑳᐧᔖᓐ ᑮᔮᐦ ᐊᓂᔮᐦ ᐊᐧᐋᔨᐤᐦ ᑳ ᐋᔨᒥᐦᐄᑯᑦ ᐅᐦᑑᑳᐦᑊᒡ ᒌᐦ ᒥᐧᑖᐦᑎᐧᐋᔨᒋᒑᓂᐦᐄ ᐅᑖᐹᓈᔅᑯᐦ ᓂᑐᐦᑯᔨᓂᑭᒥᑯᐦᑊᒡ ᒑ ᐄᔅᐱᔨᐦᐄᑯᑦ᙮ ᐋᔦᐧᐃᑯᓐᐦ ᐅᔮᐦ ᐅᐧᐹᔨᒻᐦ ᑳ ᐋᐱᔨᒡᐦ ᐊᓂᑎᐦ ᑖᐦᑎᐳᐧᐃᓂᐦᑊᒡ ᐹᔓᒡ ᐅᓂᐹᐧᐃᓂᐦᑊᒡ, ᐊᓂᔮᐦ ᑳ ᐄᑎᑯᑦ, ᐊᐧᐋᓐ ᒑ ᒌᐦ ᔮᔅᒋᐦᐄᔅᒃ ᓈᔥᒡ ᐋᐦ ᑖᐦᒋᐳᔨᓐ ᑮᔮᐦ ᐋᐦ ᒥᒋᓯᔨᓐ ᐊᓐ ᒌᔨ ᐋᓯᓈᑯᓯᔨᓐ᙮ ᒥᑯ ᐄᔑ ᐧᑳᔅᒋᓯᓐ ᐊᓂᑖᐦ ᐧᑳᔥᑖᐦ ᐋᔑᐦᒃ᙮

ᐃᔭᔅ 2007 ᑳ ᐃᒋᔥᑌᒡ ᐊᔅᒌᐤ ᐊᒋᐦᑖᓯᓐ ᒫᒃ ᐅᑌ ᐃᔑ ᐋᔥᑕᒥᑌ, ᓇᒧᐃ ᓈᔅᒡ ᐅᐦᒋ ᒥᔦᐸᔦᒡ ᐊᓂᑕ ᒉᓂᕕᕐ ᑲᐧᒑᓇᔮ ᐧᒑᐯᔅ ᐧᐄᒋᐧᐋᐧᐋᐦᑊᒡ᙮ ᐯᔫᐧᑳᐤ ᐁ ᒉᐧᑳᑎᐱᔅᑲᔨᒡ, ᒌ ᐅᑎᓇᒻ ᓂᑐᐦᑯᐃᓐᐦ, ᒥᐦᒉᑐ ᒌ ᐊᑯᐦᒋᐸᔨᐦᑖᐤ, ᑳ ᐧᐄᐧᐄᑦ ᐁᑯ ᒥᓂᐦᐧᑫᐅᑲᒥᑯᐦᑊᒡ ᑳ ᓂᑑ ᐲᐦᒉᑦ, ᑳ ᒥᓂᐦᐧᑫᑦ ᑳᐲᔥᑌᐅᐸᔨᒡ ᐃᔅᑯᑌᐧᐋᐳᔦ ᐁᑯ ᒦᓐ ᔔᒥᓈᐴᔦ ᑳ ᒥᓂᐦᐧᑫᑦ ᑲᔭ ᓃᔓᔨᒡ ᐁ ᐃᔑᓈᑯᓂᔨᐧᑳᐤ ᑳ ᒥᔅᑲᐧᐋᑲᒥᔨᐧᑳᐤ ᐃᔅᑯᑌᐧᐋᐳᐦ᙮ ᑳ ᒫᑯᓇᐦᒃ ᑳᐲᔥᑌᐅᐸᐃ ᐴᑖᔦ, ᑳ ᐲᑯᐦᑕᑖᑦ ᐊᓂᑌ ᐁ ᔫᐃᐦᑕᑳᔨᒡ ᐁᑯ ᑳ ᒫᒋᓯᓯᑦ ᓇᐦᐋᐤ ᐅᒉᔥᑌᔫᐲᐦᑊᒡ᙮ ᑳ ᑲᐅᔑᓂᑦ ᐁᑯ ᐅᑕᐦᒑᐦᑯ ᑳ ᓇᑲᑕᒥᔨᒡ ᐧᐃᔦ ᒉᐧᑳᒡ ᐁ ᐅᐦᒋᑰᓂᔨᒡ ᐊᓂᑌ ᑳ ᒫᒋᓯᓯᑦ ᐁ ᐱᒥᔑᓂᑦ ᐊᓂᑕᐦ ᐁ ᐧᐄᓂᐦᑕᑳᔨᒡ ᐊᓂᔦ ᒥᓂᐦᐧᑫᐅᑲᒥᑯᔦ᙮

ᒌ ᐊᔨᒥᐦᐄᑰ ᐊᐧᐁᔦ ᐁ ᐄᑎᑯᑦ, “ᐁᑳᐧᐃ ᒫᒌᐦ, ᒋᓂᑐᐧᐁᔨᒥᑯᒡ ᒋᑕᐧᐋᔒᒥᒡ᙮” ᒥᑯ ᒫᒃ ᐋᑦ ᐁ ᐋᔮᐧᐋᐧᑫ ᐊᐧᐋᔕ ᒫᒃ ᐁᑳ ᐋᔮᐧᐋᐧᑫ ᔖᔅ ᒌ ᐅᑎᐦᒋᐸᓂᔦ ᑫ ᒫᒌᑦ᙮ ᑖᐧᐯ ᒫᒃ ᐁᑯᓐ ᑳ ᐃᔑᓈᑯᓯᑦ᙮

ᐧᐁᓂᔥᑳᐸᔨᑦ ᒫᒃ ᑫᐧᑳᔦ ᔑᐳᑲᒨ ᐋᐦᑯᓰᐅᑲᒥᑯᐦᑊᒡ ᑳ ᐃᐦᑖᑦ᙮ ᐊᐧᐁᓐ, ᐊᓂᔦᐦ ᒫᔅᑰᒡ ᑳ ᐯᐦᑕᐧᐋᑦ ᐁ ᐊᔨᒥᐦᐄᑯᑦ ᒌ ᑖᐦᑳᐱᐦᒉᓂᒉᔨᒉᓐᐦ ᐁ ᓂᑐᐧᐁᔨᐦᑕᒥᔨᒡ ᐋᐦᑯᓰᐅᑖᐹᓂᔦ ᒉᒌ ᐹᐸᔨᓂᔨᒡ᙮ ᐅᐧᐄᐦᐧᑫᔮᒻ ᒫᒃ, ᐊᓂᔦ ᐁᒌ ᐃᑎᑯᑦ ᐁᑳ ᓈᓂᑑ ᒉ ᐅᐦᒋ ᐧᐄ ᒪᓈᐦᐆᑖᑯᑦ ᑯᑕᒃ ᐊᐧᐁᔦ ᐧᐁᓰ ᐁ ᑖᐦᒋᐳᑦ ᑲᔭ ᐁ ᒪᒋᔑᑦ, ᐁᑯᑦ ᐊᓂᑕ ᑌᐦᑖᐳᓂᐦᑊᒡ ᑳ ᐊᐱᔨᒡ ᐯᔓᒡ ᐅᓂᐯᐧᐃᓂᔨᐦᑊᒡ ᒉᓂᕕᕐ᙮ ᑳ ᐧᑫᔅᒋᔑᓐᑦ ᐧᐃᔮᐸᒫᑦ ᐊᓂᔦᐦ ᐅᐧᐄᐦᐧᑫᔮᒻ᙮

En 2007 environ, les choses n'allaient pas très bien chez Jennifer Gloria Lowpez. Un soir, elle avala des pilules, beaucoup de pilules, et alla dans un bar où elle but de la bière, puis du vin, puis du rhum et enfin de la vodka. Puis elle attrapa une bouteille de bière vide, la cassa contre le bar et se coupa en plein dans une veine. Elle s'effondra comme une poupée désarticulée. Son esprit s'éleva et laissa son corps qui saignait encore sur le sol crasseux du pub.

Quelqu'un lui disait à l'oreille : « Reste Jennifer, tes enfants ont besoin de toi ». Toutefois, enfants ou pas, il était temps de partir. Enfin, il était temps de partir.

Jennifer se réveilla à l'hôpital de Chibougamau. Quelqu'un, probablement la personne qui lui avait parlé à l'oreille, avait appelé une ambulance. Son chum, qui lui avait dit que personne ne pourrait jamais aimer une personne aussi grosse et laide que Jennifer, était assis sur la chaise près du lit. Elle se retourna sur le côté et lui tourna le dos.

French

In 2007 or so, things at Jennifer Gloria Lowpez's home were not going so great. One night she slugged back some pills, lots of pills, and went out to a bar where she drank some beer and then some wine and then some rum and then some vodka. Then she grabbed an empty beer bottle, broke it against the bar, and cut herself right across a vein. She crumpled in a heap and her spirit lifted and left her body that was still bleeding out on the grimy pub floor.

Someone was saying into her ear, "Stay Jennifer, your kids need you." But kids or no kids, it was time to go. Finally, it was time to go.

Jennifer woke up in the Chibougamau hospital. Someone, probably that person who spoke in her ear, had called an ambulance. Her boyfriend, who had told her that no one could ever love someone as fat and ugly as Jennifer, sat in the chair by the bed. She turned over on her side and faced away from him.

English

ᐋᑯᔥ ᒫ ᒌᐦ ᐄᔅᐱᔨᒡ ᐊᓐ ᑳ ᐐᐦ ᓂᐱᐦᐄᓯᔫᓐ᙮

ᒥᔕᔫᔅᑯᓂᐲᓯᒼᐦ 2010, ᑳ ᐧᐄᐦᑎᒫᑯᑦ ᒉᓂᕕᕐ ᓂᑐᐦᑯᔨᓐᐦ ᐋᐦ ᔕᑳᐅᐱᔨᑦ᙮

ᒥᒄ ᐋᔥᐱᔒᑦ ᐋᐦ ᒫᑐᑦ ᓈᐅᔥ᙮ ᒑᒁᓐ ᐊᓐ ᐋᐦ ᔕᑳᐅᐱᔨᓈᓂᐧᐃᒡ᙮ ᓂᒧᐃ ᐋ ᒑᒃ ᓂᒥ ᐧᐋᐱᐦᑎᒧᒡ ᐊᐧᐋᓂᒌ ᑮᔫᐦ ᐋᐦ ᒫᔫᑎᓂᔨᒡ ᐅᔫᐧᐋᐤᐦ ᑮᔫᐦ ᒑᒃ ᐋᑎ ᒥᓂᔑᑭᓂᐧᐃᐧᐃᔨᒡᐦ ᐹᑎᔥ ᐋᑳ ᐃᐦᑎᑯᓂᔨᒡᐦ ᓈᔥᑎᔨᒡ ᐅᔅᐱᑐᓂᐧᐋᐤᐦ ᑮᔫᐦ ᒫᒃ ᐅᔅᑳᑎᐧᐋᐤᐦ᙮ ᒨᔥ ᑳ ᐄᔑᓈᑯᓂᔨᒡᐦ ᒉᓂᕕᕐ ᐅᑑᐦᑎᓐᐦ ᐋᐦ ᐹᔑᐱᔨᔨᒡᐦ: ᐊᓐ ᒫᒃ ᐊᐧᐋᓐ ᒑ ᐧᐄᓈᔨᒡ ᐅᓯᑦ ᑮᔫᐦ ᒑᒃ ᒑ ᒥᓂᔑᑭᓂᐧᐃᐧᐃᔨᒡ, ᓂᒧᐃ ᐋᐦ ᐧᐄᔨ ᒉᓂᕕᕐ᙮ ᒑᒃ ᒦᓐ ᐊᓂᔫ ᑯᑎᒋᔨᐤ ᐅᓯᑦ, ᒦᓐ ᐊᓂᔫ ᐅᔅᐱᑐᓐ ᑮᔫᐦ ᒑᒃ ᒦᓐ ᐊᓂᔫ ᑯᑎᒋᔨᐤ ᐅᔅᐳᑐᓐ ᐋᑯᐦ ᒑᒃ ᓂᒥ ᑭᑎ ᐃᐦᑎᑯᓂᔨᐤᐦ ᐧᐋᒋᐹᔨᒄ ᐅᔅᐱᑐᓐᐦ ᑮᔫᐦ ᐅᔅᑳᑦᐦ ᑮᔫᐦ ᒑ ᐃᓯᓈᑯᓯᑦ ᒥᓯᐧᐋ ᐋᐦ ᒥᔭᐧᐃᑦ᙮

ᐊᓐ ᐋᐱᑎᓰᓰ ᑳ ᐧᐄᒋᐦᐋᑦ ᐊᐧᐋᔨᐤᐦ ᑯᐃᔅᒄ ᒑ ᒌᐦ ᐄᔑ ᒦᒋᓯᔨᒡᐦ ᐋᔭᐧᐃᑯᓐᐦ ᑳ ᐊᔨᒥᐦᐄᑯᑦ ᒉᓂᕕᕐ ᑮᔫᐦ ᒥᒄ ᒫᔨᑯᑦ ᒫᓐ ᒑᐧᑳᔨᐤ ᒑ ᑳᓯᒑᐳᐦᐅᓯᑦ ᒫᐧᑳᒡ ᐋᐦ ᒫᑐᑦ ᒥᒄ ᒫᒃ ᓂᒧᐃ ᓈᔥᒡ ᐅᐦᒋ ᐧᐋᐧᐄᐦᑎᒫᑰ ᒑᐧᑳᔨᐤ᙮ ᐋᔫᐱᒡ ᒫᒃ, ᑳ ᐅᑎᓂᐦᒃ ᐊᓂᔫᐦ ᓂᑐᐦᑯᔨᓐᐦ ᑳ ᐄᑖᑭᓂᐧᐃᑦ ᒑ ᐅᑎᓂᐦᒃ ᒉᓂᕕᕐ᙮ ᐊᐱᔒᔥ ᒌᐦ ᐊᒋᐧᐃᐱᔨᐤ, ᒥᒄ ᓂᒧᐃ ᓈᔥᒡ᙮ ᐋᔫᐱᒡ ᑳ ᐄᑎᒥᒋᐦᐅᑦ ᐋᔥᒄ ᐋᐦ ᑖᐦᒋᔨᑦ᙮ ᑮᔫᐦ ᒫᒃ ᓈᔥᒡ ᐋᐦ ᒌᐦ ᑯᔥᑎᐦᒃ ᐊᓂᔫ ᐋᐦᑯᓯᐧᐃᓂᔨᐤ ᑳ ᐄᑖᑭᓂᐧᐃᑦ ᐋᐦ ᐃᔫᑦ᙮

ᐁ ᐃᑌᔨᐦᑕᐦᒃ, ᑲᒫ ᐁᑯᔥ ᒌ ᓂᐱᐧᐋᐸᓀ ᑳᐧᐄ ᓂᐸᐦᐄᓯᔫᓐ᙮

ᐧᐄᐧᐄᒪᑲᓂᐲᓯᒼ 2010 ᑳ ᐃᒋᔥᑌᒡ ᐊᔅᒌᐤ ᐊᒋᐦᑖᓯᓐ, ᐁᑯᑦ ᑳ ᐧᐄᐦᑕᒫᑯᑦ ᐅᓂᑐᐦᑯᐃᓂᒼ ᐁ ᓰᐧᐋᑲᒥᐦᐃᐧᑫᑦ᙮

ᒌ ᒫᑑ, ᐱᔑᒄ ᒌ ᒫᑑ ᑳ ᐧᐄᐦᑕᒧᐧᐋᑲᓅᑦ ᐅᔮ᙮ ᒉᐧᑳᓐ ᒫᒃ ᐊᓐ ᐁ ᓰᐧᐋᑲᒥᐦᐧᑳᓅᐦᒡ ᑳ ᐄᓈᓅᐦᒡ ᒌ ᐃᑌᔨᐦᑕᒼ᙮ ᓇᒧᐃ ᐋ ᑫᒃ ᓇᒧᐃ ᐧᐋᐸᐦᑕᒼ ᐊᐧᐁᓐ ᐁ ᓰᐧᐋᑲᒥᐦᐧᑫᑦ ᑲᔭ ᐧᐃᔭᔅ ᐊᓂᑌ ᐁ ᒥᔮᑦ, ᒋᒥᔑᑲᓅᔮ, ᑫᒄ ᐁᐅᒄ ᐁ ᐃᔑᓈᑯᓯᑦ ᐁᑳ ᐅᔅᑳᑎᑦ ᑲᔭ ᐁᑳ ᐅᔅᐱᑐᓂᑦ᙮ ᒨᔥ ᐁᒌᐧᐄ ᐹᔥᑌᔨᐧᑳᐤ ᐅᑑᐦᑎᓐ ᒥᒍᓐ ᐁ ᑖᔅᑖᔅᒋᐸᔨᒡ ᐅᔅᑲᐃᐦ; ᐁ ᐃᐦᑖᐧᑫ ᐊᐧᐁᓐ ᑫ ᒥᐅᓂᔨᐧᑫ ᐅᓯᑦ ᑫ ᓂᑐᐧᐁᔨᐦᑖᑯᓂᔨᒡ ᒫᒃ ᑫᒌ ᒪᓂᔑᑲᓄᔨᒡ ᐧᐄ ᓈᓂᑑ ᒉᓂᕕᕐ ᐁᐅᒄ ᑫ ᐃᔅᐸᔨᑦ᙮ ᑫᒃ ᐊᓂᔮ ᑯᑕᒋᔮ ᐅᓯᑦ ᑫᓐ ᐅᔅᐱᑐᓐ ᐁᒄ ᒦᓐ ᐊᓂᔮ ᑯᑕᒋᔮ ᑫᒃ ᑫ ᐃᔑᓈᑯᓯᑦ ᐁᑳ ᒥᒍᓐ ᐊᔫᑦ ᐅᔅᑳᑦ ᑲᔭ ᐅᔅᐱᑐᓐᐦ ᐁᒄ ᒫᒃ ᑫᒃ ᑫ ᐃᔑᓇᑯᓯᑦ ᑫ ᓂᐱᑦ ᐱᔑᒄ ᐁᒌ ᒥᔮᐸᔨᑦ᙮

ᓂᔮᐦ ᓂᑐᐦᑯᐃᓂᔅᐧᑫᐤ ᑳ ᐊᔨᒥᐦᐄᑯᑦ ᐁ ᐧᐋᐧᐄᐦᑕᒫᑯᑦ ᑫ ᐃᔑ ᒦᒋᓯᑦ ᒥᐦᑫᑐ ᓰᓂᔅᑌᔨᑯᒫᐧᐃᓐᐦ ᒌ ᒦᑰ ᐱᔑᒄ ᐁᒌ ᒫᑐᑦ ᒉᓂᕕᕐ ᒥᒄ ᒫᒃ ᓇᒧᐃ ᓈᔅᒡ ᒥᔅᑕᐦᐄ ᐅᐦᒋ ᐧᐋᐧᐄᐦᑕᒫᑰ᙮ ᔫᐸᒡ ᒫᒃ ᒌ ᐅᑎᓇᒼ ᐊᓂᔮᐦ ᓂᑐᐦᑯᐃᓇᐦ ᑳ ᒥᔫᑲᓅᑦ ᑫ ᐅᑎᓇᐦᒃ᙮ ᐊᐱᔒᔥ ᒌ ᐊᒎᐸᔨᐦᐄᑰ ᐊᓂᔮᐦ ᓂᑐᐦᑯᐃᓇᐦ, ᓇᒧᐃ ᒥᒄ ᓈᔅᒡ ᒥᔅᑕᐦᐄ᙮ ᔫᐸᒡ ᒌ ᒨᔑᐦᑖᐤ ᓈᔅᒡ ᐁ ᒥᓯᒋᔥᑎᑦ᙮ ᒌ ᔅᒋᐦᐄᑰ ᒫᒃ ᐅᔮ᙮

Si seulement le suicide avait fonctionné.

If only the suicide had worked.

En janvier 2010, le médecin dit à Jennifer qu'elle était diabétique.

In January 2010, the doctor told Jennifer she had diabetes.

Elle pleura, pleura, pleura. C'était quoi le diabète de toute façon ? Les personnes diabétiques ne devenaient-elles pas aveugles et ne souffraient-elles pas d'infections, puis ne subissaient-elles pas amputation après amputation jusqu'à ce qu'il ne leur reste plus de bras ou de jambes ? Les talons de Jennifer étaient toujours fissurés : si un pied devait s'infecter et être scié, ce serait le sien. Et puis ce serait au tour de son autre pied, puis un bras et puis l'autre, et bientôt elle n'aurait plus de membres et mourrait d'une mort horrible remplie de pus.

She cried and cried and cried. What was diabetes anyways? Didn't people with diabetes go blind and get infections and then amputation after amputation until they didn't have any arms or legs left? Jennifer's heels were always cracked: if anyone's foot was gonna get infected and have to be sawed off, it'd be hers. And then it'd be her other foot and then one arm and then the other and soon she wouldn't have any limbs and would die a horrible pus-filled death.

La nutritionniste qui parla du diabète à Jennifer ne cessait de lui tendre des kleenex pour assécher ses larmes, mais elle ne lui expliqua vraiment grand-chose. Malgré tout, Jennifer commença à prendre des pilules contre le diabète parce qu'elle était supposée le faire. Elles lui firent perdre quelques livres, mais pas beaucoup. Elle se sentait encore comme un arbre de Noël. Un arbre de Noël terrifié.

The nutritionist who talked to Jennifer about diabetes kept handing her Kleenex for her tears but didn't really explain much. Still, Jennifer started taking diabetes pills because she was supposed to. They made her lose a few pounds, but not many. She still felt like a Christmas tree. A terrified Christmas tree.

ᒥᒄ ᒫᒃ ᒌᐦ ᐃᐦᑎᑯᓂᔭᐤ ᒑᐧᑳᔭᐤ ᐋᐦ ᒌᐦ ᐄᑖᔭᐦᑎᐦᒃ ᐋᐦ ᐧᐄᒋᐦᐄᑯᑦ ᐋᔑᑯᒥᒌᔑᑳᐤᐦ᙮ ᓂᔥᐧᑖᐤ ᐋᐦ ᒦᑎᓯᑦ ᐹᔭᑯᒌᔑᑳᐤᐦ ᑭᔮᐦ ᓃᔓ ᐧᒑᑭᓚᑦᐦ, ᐋᔭᐦᑯᓈᔥᐦ ᑭᔮᐦ ᐴᑏᓐ ᐋᐦ ᓯᓈᑭᐧᐃᑦ, ᑭᔮᐦ ᓈᔥᒡ ᐋᐦ ᒥᐦᒋᐧᐃᑖᔭᔭᒡᐦ ᒋᐸᔅ ᑭᔮᐦ ᐋᐦ ᐋᑯᐦᒋᒧᑦ ᒑᐧᑳᔭᐤ ᑭᔮᐦ ᓃᔓ ᐱᐧᔮᐳᔅᑯᔮᑭᓐ ᑳ ᔒᐧᐋᑮᒥᔑᔭᒡ ᐋᐦ ᐧᐄᒋᐦᐄᑯᑦ ᐅᑎᐧᐋᔑᔒᒻᐦ, ᑭᔮᐦ ᑯᐧᑖᔥᒡ ᑎᐦᑐ ᑳᐲᔥᒑᐅᐲᔑᔭᒡ ᑭᔮᐦ ᐹᔭᒄ ᑭᔮᐦ ᒫᒃ ᓃᔓᒥᓂᐦᐧᑳᑭᓐ ᔔᒥᓈᐳᔭᐤ ᑭᔮᐦ ᒑᒃ ᑳ ᒌ ᒋᑖᑦ ᐧᐋᑖᑯᔔᒦᑎᓯᐧᑖᐤᐦ ᑭᔮᐦ ᐋᑎ ᑎᐱᔅᑳᔭᒡᐦ ᑳᐦ ᑰᔑᒧᔭᒡᐦ ᐅᑎᐧᐋᔑᔒᒻᐦ᙮ ᒦᓐ ᒫᒃ, ᐋᔑᒧᒻ ᒥᑖᐦᑐᒌᔑᑳᐤᐦ, ᑳ ᒌ ᒥᓂᐦᐧᑳᑦ ᒉᓂᕕᕐ ᒥᑎᑑᓐ ᓃᔓᒌᔑᑳᐤᐦ ᐋᑳ ᐴᓃᑦ᙮ ᓈᔥᒡ ᐋᑳ ᐅᐦᒋ ᒥᐧᔮᔭᐦᑎᒥᔭᒡᐦ ᐊᓂᔮᐦ ᐅᑎᐧᐋᔑᔒᒻᐦ, ᒥᒄ ᒫᒃ ᒉᓂᕕᕐ ᒌᐦ ᐧᐄᐦ ᒥᐧᔮᔭᐦᑎᒥᐦᐄᓰ, ᑭᔮᐦ ᓂᒥ ᐅᐦᒋ ᐧᐄ ᒋᔅᒋᓰᑎᑎᒻ ᒑᐧᑳᔭᐤ᙮ ᑭᔮᐦ ᐊᓂᔮ ᑯᑫᐃᓐ ᐋᔨᐧᐃᒄ ᒦᓐ ᑳ ᒌ ᐋᐱᒋᐦᑖᑦ᙮ ᓂᐧᐄᒋᐦᐄᑯᓐ ᐋᐦ ᒌᐦ ᐄᑖᔭᐦᑎᐦᒃ᙮ ᐄᐦᐄ, ᑖᐧᐹᐦ ᓂᐧᐄᒋᐦᐄᑯᓐ ᑯᑫᐃᓐ ᒌᐦ ᐄᑖᔭᐦᑎᒻ᙮ ᐋᔨᐧᐃᒄ ᑳ ᒌ ᐋᐱᒋᐦᑖᑦ ᓃᐧᔔᔥᒡ ᑭᔮᐦ ᒫᒃ ᓂᔮᓈᓈᐤ ᑎᐦᐧᑖᐤ ᐹᔭᑯᑎᐧᐃᔥᑖᐤᐦ᙮

ᐹᑎᒫᐦ ᒫᒃ ᐊᓂᔮ ᑳ ᐧᐄᐦᑎᒧᐧᐋᑭᓂᐧᐃᑦ ᐋᐦ ᔔᑳᐅᐱᔭᑦ, ᑳ ᓰᑯᓂᔭᒡ 2011 ᑳ ᐄᒋᔥᑖᔭᒡ ᐋᐦ ᐱᐳᓂᔭᒡ, ᐊᓂᑖᐦ ᒥᓖᓐᓛᓐ ᐋᑯᑖᐦ ᑳ ᐄᔅᐱᔭᒡ ᒉᓂᕕᕐ ᐋᐦ ᐹᔭᑯᑖᐅᓰᒡ ᑭᔮᐦ ᑳ ᓃᐳᐧᐃᑦ ᐊᓂᑖᐦ ᐋᐦ ᓃᐱᑖᐳᐧᐃᓈᓂᐧᐃᐧᐃᔭᒡ ᐋᐦ ᐋᓯᓂᐧᐋᓯᑦ ᒑ ᐱᐹᒥᐱᔭᑦ᙮ ᐊᓂᑎᐦ ᓃᑳᓂᐦᒡ ᐋᐦ ᐄᐦᑖᑦ ᐋᑯᑎᐦ ᓈᐳᐧᐃᔭᒡᐦ ᐊᓂᔮᐦ ᐅᐧᐹᔭᒻᐦ ᐋᐦ ᐱᐹᐦᐱᐦᐋᔭᒡᐦ ᐊᓂᔮᐦ ᐅᑎᐧᐋᔑᔒᒥᐧᐋᐤᐦ ᒫᐧᑳᒡ ᐊᓂᑎᐦ ᐋᐦ ᓃᐳᐧᐃᒡ, ᑳᓂᐧᐋᐱᒫᑦ ᒉᓂᕕᕐ ᑭᔮᐦ ᐊᐧᑳᑖᔭᐦᑎᐦᒃ᙮ ᒑᑲᑦ

ᒌ ᐃᐦᑕᑯᓂᔩ ᑮᐹ ᑫᐧᑳᔩ ᒣᔑᑯᒻ ᒌᔑᑳᐤ ᐁ ᒥᔦᔭᐦᑕᒥᐦᐄᑯᑦ᙮ ᓂᔥᐧᑖᐤ ᒌ ᒦᑎᓰ ᐯᔭᒄ ᒌᔑᑳᐤ ᑲᔦ ᓃᔓ ᐧᒑᑲᓚᑦ ᒌ ᒦᒎ ᑲᔦ ᐋᐦᐃᑯᓈᔅ ᑲᔦ ᒫᒃ ᐴᒌᓐ ᑕᐦᐧᑖᐤ ᐁ ᓰᐧᐁᔩᒪᐦᒋᐦᐅᑦ, ᓀᔅᑕ ᑲᔦ ᒣᔑᑯᒻ ᐅᑖᑯᓰᐦ ᑳ ᑳᔅᐱᑌᔭᐧᑳᐤ ᐸᑌᑎᔅ ᒌᑰ ᐊᔅᐸᔅᑕᒫᐧᐃᓂᔩ ᒌ ᒦᒎᒡ ᐅᑕᐧᐋᔒᒻᐦ, ᑲᔦ ᓃᔓ ᑳᐧᐄᐹᑲᒥᔭᒡ ᑳᓰᐧᐋᑲᒥᔑᔭᐧᑳᐤᐦ ᒌ ᒥᓂᐦᐧᑫᐅᒡ, ᑲᔦ ᒫᒃ ᑯᐧᑖᔅᒡ ᑳ ᐲᔥᑌᐅᐸᔭᔭᐧᑳᐤ ᓀᔅᑕ ᐯᔭᒄ ᒫᒃ ᓃᔓ ᒥᓂᐦᐧᑳᑲᓐ ᔔᒥᓈᐳᔩ ᒌ ᒥᓂᐦᐧᑫᐤ ᒫᒋᓯᒡ, ᑳ ᑰᔑᒧᔭᒡ ᐅᑕᐧᐋᔒᒻ ᐁᔅᒄ ᒌ ᒥᓂᐦᐧᑫᐤ᙮ ᑕᐦᐧᑖᐤ ᒥᐦᑖᐦᑐ ᒌᔑᑳᐤ ᐧᐁᑎᐦᒋᐸᔭᔭᒡ ᒫᒃ ᐅᔥᑌ ᒥᑖᐦᑐ, ᐁᒄ ᐱᔑᒄ ᑳᒌ ᒥᓂᐦᐧᑫᑦ ᓃᔓ ᒌᔑᑳᐤᐦ ᐃᔥᐱᔥ᙮ ᓇᒧᐃ ᒥᒍᓐ ᐅᐦᒋ ᒥᔦᔭᐦᑕᒥᔩ ᐅᑕᐧᐋᔒᒻᐦ ᐅᔩ ᐁ ᐃᐦᑎᑦ, ᒌ ᓂᑐᐧᐁᔭᐦᑕᒻ ᒉᓂᕕᕐ ᒉᒌ ᐄᒉᐸᔭᔭᒡ ᑖᓐ ᑳ ᐃᑕᒪᐦᒋᐦᐅᑦ ᐁᐅᒄ ᐧᐁᐦᒌ ᒥᓂᐦᐧᑫᑦ, ᒌ ᓂᑐᐧᐁᔭᐦᑕᒻ ᑫᐧᑳᔩ ᑫ ᐧᐄᒋᐦᐄᑯᑦ᙮ ᐁᔩ ᒫᒃ ᐧᑳᑫᐃᓐ ᒌ ᐃᐦᑑᑕᒻ ᐊᓂᔩ ᑳ ᐧᐋᐹᔭᒡ ᒪᒋᓂᑐᐦᑯᐃᓂᔩ᙮ ᓂᐧᐄᒋᐦᐄᑰᓐ ᒌ ᐃᑌᔭᐦᑕᒻ ᐊᓂᔩ ᐁ ᐅᑎᓇᐦᒃ᙮ ᐧᐃᔦᔅ ᓃᐧᔔᐧᔔᐤ ᒫᒃ ᓂᔮᓈᓀᐧᐋᐤ ᒌ ᐃᐦᑑᑕᒻ ᐅᔩ ᐯᔭᒄ ᑑᔥᑌᐤᐦ᙮

ᓇᒧᐃ ᒥᐦᑫᑐ ᐲᓯᒻ ᐊᓂᑕ ᐅᐦᒋ ᑳ ᐧᐄᐦᑕᒧᐧᐋᑲᓅᒡ ᐁ ᓰᐧᐋᑲᒥᐦᐧᑫᒡ, ᐁ ᓰᑯᓂᔭᒡ 2011 ᐊᔅᒌᐤ ᐊᒋᐦᑖᓯᓂᔩ, ᒪᓖᓐᓛᓐᑦ ᒌ ᐃᔅᐸᔩᒡ ᐁ ᐯᔭᑯᑌᐅᓰᐧᑖᐤ᙮ ᑳ ᓃᐳᐧᑖᐤ ᐊᓂᑕ ᐁ ᐊᔓᐧᐋᐱᐧᑖᐤ ᑫᒌ ᐴᔑᐧᑖᐤ ᑳ ᒑᐦᒌᓂᐧᑳᐸᔭᔭᒡ᙮ ᐅᐦᒋᔥᑰ ᐊᓂᑕ ᐁ ᐃᐦᑖᑦ ᒌ ᓃᐳᔩᐦ ᐅᐧᐄᐦᐧᑫᔮᒻ, ᐁ ᒨᒋᑲᐦᐋᑦ ᐊᓂᔩᐦ ᐊᐧᐋᔓ ᐊᓂᑕ ᑳ ᓈᓃᐳᔭᐧᑖᐤ, ᐁ ᒫᒥᑐᓀᔭᐦᑕᐦᒃ ᒉᓂᕕᕐ ᐊᓂᔩ ᐁ ᐃᔑᑳᐳᑦ ᐁ ᑲᓇᐧᐋᐸᒫᑦ᙮ ᒫᓐᐦ ᐅᔔ ᐧᐋᐦᐁᔩ ᒌ ᐋᐸᑎᓯᔩᐦ

Ce qui était bien, c'était le réconfort apporté tous les jours. Trois repas, plus deux tablettes de chocolat par jour, auxquels s'ajoutaient des biscuits et de la poutine entre les repas, plus un gros sac de chips avec trempette de chez Costco et deux bouteilles de Pepsi avec ses enfants chaque soir, en plus d'un pack de six bières et d'un ou deux verres de vin qu'elle vidait graduellement au cours du souper et tout au long de la soirée après que les enfants soient allés au lit. Et puis, tous les dix jours environ, Jennifer buvait à l'excès pour se remettre d'aplomb et être soûle pendant deux journées complètes. Les excès de boisson dérangeaient ses enfants, mais Jennifer avait besoin de réconfort, d'évasion. Oh, et la cocaïne. La cocaïne la faisait définitivement se sentir mieux. Elle la faisait se sentir mieux environ sept ou huit fois par semaine.

Quelques mois après son diagnostic du diabète, au printemps 2011, Jennifer alla avec sa famille à Marineland. Elle faisait la queue avec sa famille pour manège. Son chum se tenait devant elle et plaisantait avec les enfants qui faisaient la queue. Jennifer le regardait et réfléchissait. Il était au travail la moitié du temps et il était vraiment séduisant. Même après avoir été ensemble par intermittence

The good thing was that comfort was available every single day. Three meals plus two chocolate bars a day, plus snacks of cookies and poutine between meals, plus a big Costco bag of chips and dip along with a couple of bottles of Pepsi with her kids every night, plus a six-pack of beer and a glass or two of wine gradually emptied over dinner and through the evening after the kids had gone to bed. And then, every ten days or so, Jennifer would binge-drink to get good and wasted for two solid days. The bingeing bugged her kids, but Jennifer needed comfort, escape. Oh, and cocaine. Cocaine definitely made her feel better. It made her feel better about seven or eight times a week.

A few months after her diabetes diagnosis, in spring of 2011, Jennifer went with her family to Marineland and stood in line with them to go on a ride. Her boyfriend was standing in front of her, joking with the kids in line, and Jennifer was looking him over and thinking. He was gone at work half the time and he was hot. Even after eighteen years of being together on and off, he was hot. It

ᒨᔥ ᓂᒥ ᐃᐦᑖᐤ ᐋᐦ ᐋᐱᑎᓰᑦ ᒥᑯ ᒫᒃ ᓈᔥᒡ ᐋᐦ ᒥᐧᔮᐹᐅᔑᑦ᙮ ᐋᑦ ᔖᔥ ᓂᔮᓈᓈᐅᔖᑉ ᑎᐦᑐᐱᐳᓐᐦ ᒑᑲᑦ ᒨᔥ ᐋᐦ ᒌᐦ ᐧᐄᒑᐧᐋᑦ, ᐋᔮᐱᒡ ᐋᔥᑯ ᓈᔥᒡ ᒌᐦ ᒥᔪᓂᐧᐋᐤ᙮ ᓈᔥᒡ ᐋᐦ ᒌᐦ ᒥᔪᐧᐃᓂᐧᐋᑦ ᐊᓂᔮ ᐋᐦ ᐱᒋᔅᑭᓈᐱᔨᒡᐦ ᐋᔪᐧᐃᑯ ᐊᓂᔮ ᓈᔥᒡ ᑳ ᒥᔪᐧᐃᓂᐧᒫᑦ᙮

ᒥᑯ ᒫᒃ ᓈᔥᒡ ᐋᐦ ᒌᐦ ᒥᔨᒑᔨᒫᑦ᙮ ᓈᔥᒡ ᐄᔨᐦᒡ ᐋᐦ ᒌᐦ ᐄᑖᔨᒫᑦ ᑭᔮᐦ ᒨᔮᒻ ᓈᔥᒡ ᐋ̈ᑲ ᒨᔮᒻ ᐄᑖᔨᒫᑦ ᑭᔮᐦ ᒨᔮᒻ ᐊᓂᑖᐦ ᓈᓈᓂᒌᒻ ᐋᐦ ᐧᐄᐦ ᑭᑳᑖᔨᒡᐦ ᒑᐧᑳᔨᐤ: ᒌᐦ ᐊᑖᒫᔨᒫᐤ ᑫᓂᔑᔅᐦ ᑯᑎᒃᐦ ᐊᐧᐋᔨᐤᐦ ᐋᐦ ᐧᐄᒑᐧᐋᔨᒡᐦ, ᓈᔥᒡ ᐋᐦ ᒌᐦ ᑯᔥᐧᑳᔨᒫᑦ ᑫᓂᔑᔅ, ᐋᔪᐧᐃᑯ ᐋᑯᐦ ᐊᓂᔮ ᐋᐦ ᒌᐦ ᐄᑎᑯᑦ ᒫᓐᐦ ᐋ̈ᑲ ᓂᐦᑖ ᒑ ᐃᐦᑖᔨᒡᐦ ᐊᐧᐋᔨᐤᐦ ᐋᐦ ᓂᑎᐧᐋᐦᔨᒥᑯᑦ = ᐋᑯᐦ ᐋᑖᔨᐦᑎᐦᒃ ᑖᓂᑖᐦ ᒑ ᒌᐦ ᐅᐦᒋ ᐧᐄᒑᐧᐃᒃ ᑯᑎᒃ ᐊᐧᐋᓐ᙮ ᑭᔮᐦ ᐊᓂᔮᐦ ᐅᑖᓂᓯᐧᐋᐤᐦ ᓈᔥᒡ ᐄᔨᐦᒡ ᐋᐦ ᒌᐦ ᐃᐦᑎᔨᒡᐦ ᑭᔮᐦ ᒨᔮᒻ ᐋᐦ ᐧᐄᐦ ᑭᑳᑖᔨᒡ ᑭᔮᐦ ᒑᐧᑳᔨᐤ᙮ ᒥᓯᐧᐋ ᒑᐧᑳᔨᐤ ᓈᔥᒡ ᐄᔨᐦᒡ ᐋᐦ ᒌᐦ ᐄᑖᔨᐦᑖᑯᓂᔨᒡ ᑭᔮᐦ ᓈᔥᒡ ᐋ̈ᑲ ᐅᐦᒋ ᒌᐦ ᒥᔪᔥᑳᑐᒡ᙮ ᓈᓂᑑ ᐧᐋᔥ ᒑᐧᑳᓐ ᐄᔅᐱᔨᒋᒑ ᐄᑖᔨᐦᑎᒻ ᑫᓂᔑᔅ᙮

ᒑᒃ ᑳ ᐅᑎᐦᒋᐳᔨᒡ ᒑ ᐱᐹᒥᐱᔨᒡ ᑭᔮᐦ ᐊᓂᑖᐦ ᐋᔑ ᐴᓯᑦ ᑫᓂᔑᔅ ᑭᔮᐦ ᐋᑎ ᐅᐧᐋᔨᐱᑦ = ᒥᑯ ᓂᒥ ᒌᔨᐧᐋ ᒌᐦ ᒫᑯᐱᑏᓰ᙮ ᐊᓂᔮ ᑭᔨᐧᐹ ᓈᔥᒡ ᐋᐦ ᒥᓯᒋᔅᑎᒃ, ᒥᓯᐧᐋ ᐊᐧᐋᔨᐤᐦ ᐧᐃᔮᐱᑯᑦ, ᐋ̈ᑲ ᐅᐦᒋ ᒌᐦ ᒫᑯᐱᑏᓯᑦ᙮

ᒫᓐᐦ ᒥᐧᔮᐯᐤ ᒌ ᐃᑌᔨᒉᐤ ᑲᔦ᙮ ᐋᑦ ᒫᒃ ᔮᔅ ᓂᔮᓈᓀᐅᔖᑉ ᐱᐳᓐᐦ ᑳ ᐃᔥᐱᔥ ᒋᔅᒉᔨᒥᑐᐧᑖᐤ ᐋᔥᑰ ᒥᑯ ᐁ ᐧᐄᒉᐅᑐᐧᑖᐤ, ᐁᔅᑯ ᒌ ᒨᔥᑌᓇᐧᐁᐤ᙮ ᒌ ᐧᐋᔐᑲᒥᑐᐧᐋᐱᔫ ᐁᐅᑯ ᐊᓂᔫᐦ ᐅᔅᒌᔑᑯᔫᐦ ᓈᔅᒡ ᑳ ᒦᐅᓇᒧᐧᐋᑦ᙮

ᒌ ᒨᔑᐦᐧᐁᐤ ᐋᐦᒌᐅᐦ ᐁ ᐃᐦᑌᔨᐦᑖᑯᓯᔨᒡ᙮ ᐃᔅᑲ ᐧᐁᑖᒡ ᐧᐃ ᒋᔅᑳᔦᔨᐦᑕᒥᔫᐧᐋᐦ ᒌ ᐃᐦᑎᔫᐦ ᑲᔦ ᒧᐧᐁᒡ ᐁ ᑳᑖᑦ ᑫᐧᑳᔫ ᒌ ᐃᑌᔨᒉᐤ; ᒌ ᐋᓄᒉᐤ ᑫᓂᔑᔅᐦ ᐁ ᐄᑖᑦ ᑯᑕᒃ ᐊᐧᐁᔫᐦ ᐁ ᐧᐄᑫᐧᐋᔨᒡ ᒥᑯ ᒫᒃ ᑖᓂᑌ ᑫᒌ ᐅᐦᒋ ᐃᐦᑎᔮᓐ ᐊᓐ ᒌ ᐃᑌᔨᐦᑕᒻ ᑫᓂᔑᔅ ᐁᒌ ᐃᑎᑯᑦ ᑮᐹ ᐁᑳ ᐧᐄᔅᑳᒡ ᑯᑕᒃ ᐊᐧᐁᔫᐦ ᑫ ᐅᐦᒋ ᓂᑐᐧᐁᔨᒥᑯᑦ = ᑖᓂᑌ ᒫᒃ ᑫᒌ ᐅᐦᒋ ᑯᑕᒃ ᐊᐧᐁᔫᐦ ᐧᐄᑫᐅᒪᒡ ᒌ ᐃᑌᔨᐦᑕᒻ᙮ ᐊᓂᔫ ᒫᒃ ᐅᑖᓂᓯᐧᐋᐤ ᓈᔅᒡ ᐋᐦᒌᐅᐦ ᐁᒌ ᐃᑌᔨᐦᑖᑯᓯᔨᒡ ᒧᐧᐁᔥᒡ ᑫᐧᑳᔫ ᐁ ᑳᑖᔨᒡ ᐁ ᐃᐦᑎᔨᒡ᙮ ᒌ ᐅᔥᑕᐧᐁᔨᐦᑕᒥᐦᐄᑯ ᑲᔦ ᓇᒧᐃ ᐅᐦᒋ ᓇᐦᐄᔥᑲᑯ ᑫᐧᑳᔫ᙮ ᒌ ᒨᔑᐦᑖᐤ ᑫᐧᑳᔫ ᐁ ᐃᔅᐸᔨᔨᒡ᙮

ᑫᒃ ᑳ ᐅᑎᐦᑕᐦᐧᑳᐤ ᐊᓂᑌ ᑫ ᐅᐦᒋ ᐴᔑᐧᑖᐤ ᑳ ᐸᐸ̈ᒫᐱᐦᑫᐸᔨᔨᒡ ᐁᑯ ᑳᐧᐄ ᐧᐊᐧᐁᔭᐱᑦ ᐊᓂᑕ ᐁ ᐊᐱᓈᓅᔨᒡ = ᓇᒧᐃ ᐅᐦᒌ ᒋᐸᐦᐄᐸᓂᔫ ᐊᓂᔫ ᒋᐹᔅᑯᐦᐄᑲᓂᔫ ᐊᓂᑕ ᐅᔅᐱᔅᑯᓂᐦᒡ᙮ ᐅᔖᑲᓂᐦᒡ ᐁᑯᑦ ᑳ ᓇᑳᐦᑎᓂᔨᒡ ᐧᐁᓵ ᐁ ᒥᓯᒋᔥᑎᑦ, ᒥᓯᐧᐁ ᒫᒃ ᐊᐧᐁᔫᐦ ᐁ ᑲᓇᐧᐋᐸᒥᑯᑦ, ᐊᓂᔫ ᑮᐹ ᐁᑳ ᒌ ᐴᔑᑦ ᐧᐁᓵ ᐁ ᑖᐦᒋᐳᑦ᙮

depuis dix-huit ans, il était séduisant. Ses yeux bleus étaient ce qui changeaient la donne.

was his blue eyes that did it.

Toutefois, il se passait quelque chose de bizarre. Ces jours-ci, il était encore plus lunatique, étrange et secret que d'habitude : il avait accusé Jennifer de le tromper, ce qui était la chose la plus ridicule au monde, car, comme il le faisait parfois remarquer, personne ne voudrait jamais d'elle – donc, franchement, comment pourrait-elle le tromper ? Et leur fille agissait également de façon étrange et secrète. Tout en était gênant et inconfortable. Quelque chose se tramait.

But something weird was going on. These days he was acting even more moody and strange and secretive than usual: he had accused Jennifer of cheating on him which was the most ridiculous thing in the world because, as he sometimes pointed out, no one would ever want her – so, you know, how could she cheat? And their daughter was acting strange and secretive too. Everything was awkward and uncomfortable all around. Something was up.

Leur tour pour le manège arriva et Jennifer entra dans l'enclos pour s'asseoir dans son siège. Toutefois, la barrière du manège ne pouvait pas se verrouiller derrière elle. Elle cognait sur son cul d'arbre de Noël qui était, comme tout le monde pouvait le voir, trop gros pour le manège.

Their turn at the ride came and Jennifer stepped into the enclosure to sit in her seat – but the ride gate couldn't latch behind her. It just banged into her Christmas tree ass which was, for everyone there to see, obviously too fat for the ride.

“ᓂᒥᐦᒌᐧᐋᓯᓐ,” ᐄᑎᑰ ᐊᓂᔮᐦ ᑳ ᐱᒥᐱᔨᐦᑖᔨᒡᐦ ᐹᐦᑳᒡ᙮ “ᑖᐹ ᓂᓂᑎᐧᐋᔨᐦᑖᑯᓯᓈᓐ ᒑ ᐴᓯᐦᐄᒋᐦᑦ ᐊᐧᐋᓐ ᐚᑲ ᒫᑯᐱᓯᑦ᙮ ᒥᒄ ᒫᒃ ᐊᓂᑖᐦ ᐄᔑ ᔖᑭᒋᐧᐋᔨᓈ,” ᓈᑖᐦ ᐋᔑ ᐊᑐᐦᐄᒑᔨᒡᐦ ᐄᔥᐱᒥᐦᒡ ᐊᓂᑎᐦ ᒑ ᒋᐱᐦᒋᐱᔨᔨᒡ, “ᐋᑯᑖᐦ ᓈᑖᐦ ᒑ ᒌᐦ ᔑᓂᐧᐋᐦᐄᐧᑖᐤ ᐊᓂᒌ ᑭᐹᐧᑖᐧᐋ᙮”

ᑯᐃᔅᒄ ᑭᔮᐦ ᐹᐦᑳᒡ ᒌ ᐊᔨᒥᐦᐄᑰ᙮

ᓂᔮᒥᔅᐧᑳᔨᑦ ᒉᓂᕕᕝ, ᐊᓂᑖᐦ ᐋᔑ ᓃᐦᑎᒋᐧᐋᑦ ᐊᓂᑎᐦ ᑳᐦ ᐊᐱᑦ, ᑭᔮᐦ ᐋᑎ ᔖᑭᒋᐧᐋᑦ ᓈᑖᐦ ᐄᔥᐱᒥᐦᒡ ᒑ ᐊᔑᓂᐧᐋᐦᐋᑦ᙮ ᓈᔥᒡ ᐋᐦ ᒌᐦ ᐅᐧᐋᓂᐦᑎᒋᑦ᙮

ᑭᔨᐧᐹ ᑖᐧᐹᐦ, ᓈᔥᑖᐧᐹᐦ ᒌ ᐃᔮᔨᒦᔨᑰ ᒑ ᒌᐦ ᐃᔮᔮᐦᒌᑦ = ᒥᒄ ᐋᐦ ᑭᓂᐧᐋᐱᐦᑎᐦᒃ ᐋᐦ ᐱᔅᑯᑖᐅᐦᑳᔨᒡ ᑭᔮᐦ ᐋᐦ ᐄᑖᔨᐦᑎᐦᒃ ᒑ ᔖᑭᒋᐧᐊᑦ ᒌᐦ ᒨᐦᐄᑰ᙮ ᑭᔨᐧᐹ ᑖᐧᐹᐦ, ᒌ ᒥᓯᒋᔅᑎᐤ = ᒌᐦ ᐅᔑᓈᓲ ᑭᔮᐦ ᓂᒥ ᐅᐦᒋ ᔖᐧᑳᔨᒨ ᒑ ᒌᐦ ᐧᐄᐦᑎᐦᒃ ᓈᔥᒡ ᐋᐦ ᐧᐋᔅᒻ ᒥᓯᒋᔅᑎᒃ᙮ ᐋᑯᑖᐦ ᐋᓯᓈᑯᓯᑦ ᐊᐧᐋᓐ ᔖᔥ ᐋᐦ ᐅᑎᐧᐋᔑᔒᒥᑦ ᐋᐦ ᓂᔮᓈᓈᐅᔖᐳᐳᐧᓈᓯᑦ ᑭᔮᐦ ᐚᑲ ᐴᓃᑦ ᐋᐦ ᐅᑎᐧᐋᔑᔒᒥᑦ, ᒫᒃ ᐋᑎ ᓈᐅᐧᐃᔨᒡᐦ, ᐅᑎᐧᐋᔑᔒᒻᐦ ᑭᔮᐦ ᒫᒃ ᐋᐦ ᐋᐱᑎᓰᑦ ᐊᓂᑎᐦ ᒫ ᒌᐦ ᐅᐦᒋ ᐱᒥᓈᑦ ᑭᔮᐦ ᐊᓂᑎᐦ ᐧᐋᔅᑲ ᐋᐦ ᐄᐦᑖᑦ ᒨᔥ ᐱᔑᔑᒄ ᐋᐦ ᐧᐋᐱᐦᑎᐦᒃ ᒫᐧᑳᔨᐤ ᒫ ᒌᐦ ᒦᒋᑦ, ᑭᔮᐦ ᐋᐦ ᒦᒋᑦ, ᓈᔥᒡ ᑭᔨᐧᐹ ᐋᐦ ᐃᔮᐧᐃᔨᔅᒡ ᐊᓂᒌ ᐊᔥᑎᐧᐋᔑᔒᒥᒡ ᐋᐦ ᒋᒋᓂᐧᑖᐤ ᑭᔮᐦ ᐚᑲ ᐄᔥᐱᔒᐦᑭᐧᐃᐧᑖᐤ᙮ ᐄᐦᐄ, ᐄᐦᐄ, ᓂᔥᐧᑖᐤ ᒥᑖᐦᑐᒥᑎᓂᐤ ᐊᐦᑐᑎᐹᐹᔥᑯᒋᑭᓈᓲ ᑭᔮᐦ

“ᓂᒥᐦᒌᐧᐁᓯᓐ, ᐃᔅᐧᑫᐤ, ᒌ ᐄᑎᑰ ᐊᓂᔫᐦ ᑳ ᓇᓈᑲᒋᐦᑖᔨᒡ ᐊᓂᑕ ᐁ ᐴᔑᓈᓄᔨᒡ ᒋᔮᒻ ᐁ ᐊᔨᒥᐦᐄᑯᑦ, “ᓇᒧᐃ ᒋᑲᒌ ᐴᔑᓐ ᐁᐅᒄ ᐁ ᐃᒋᔥᑌᒡ ᓂᐧᐄᔐᐧᐁᐧᐃᓂᓈᓐ᙮ ᓄᑌ ᒫᒃ ᐃᑐᐦᑌᐦ᙮” ᐁ ᐊᑐᐦᐊᒫᑯᒡ ᓄᑌ ᐁ ᐅᐦᒋ ᑲᐹᓄᔨᒡ ᐊᓂᔫᐦ ᑳᐸᐹᒫᐱᐦᒉᐸᔨᔨᒡ, “ᐁᑯᑌ ᓄᑌ ᐊᔕᐧᐋᐸᒥᒡ ᒉ ᐃᔥᐱᔥ ᑲᐹᐧᑖᐤ ᐊᓂᒌ ᑳ ᐧᐄᒉᐅᔥᐧᑳᐤ,” ᐄᑎᑰ᙮

ᒌ ᒥᔫᐦᑖᑯᓯᔫᐦ ᑲᔦ ᒋᔮᒻ ᒌ ᐊᔨᒥᐦᐄᑰ᙮

ᑳ ᓈᓈᒥᔅᐧᑫᔨᑦ ᒉᓂᕕᕝ, ᑳ ᐄᒋᔑᑦ ᐊᓂᑕ ᑳ ᓃᐴᑦ ᐁᒄ ᑳ ᐃᑐᐦᑌᑦ ᓄᑌ ᒉ ᐅᐦᒋ ᑲᐹᔨᒡ ᐅᐯᔭᑯᑌᐅᔒᒻ᙮ ᑲᒫ ᓯᔅᒋᑰᒡ ᐁᑳ ᐃᐦᑖᔭᓐ ᐅᑕ ᒌ ᐃᑌᔨᐦᑕᒻ᙮

ᑖᐧᐯ ᑮᐹ, ᒌ ᐋᔨᒨ ᐁᐧᐄ ᐋᔮᐦᒌᑦ = ᒌ ᒫᑑ ᒫᓐᐦ ᐋᑦ ᒥᒄ ᐁ ᑲᓇᐧᐋᐸᐦᑕᐦᒃ ᐁ ᐱᔅᑯᑖᐅᐦᑳᔨᒡ ᐁ ᒋᔅᒉᔨᐦᑕᐦᒃ ᒉ ᐋᔨᒥᐦᐄᑯᑦ ᒉᒌ ᔅᑲᒋᐧᐁᑦ᙮ ᒌ ᒥᓯᒋᔥᑑ ᑖᐧᐯ = ᐧᐄᔭ ᒫᐅᒡ ᒌ ᒋᒍᐧᐁᐱᑕᒻ ᐁ ᐹᐦᐱᑦ ᒫᓐᐦ ᐅᔕᑲᓐ ᐅᐦᒋ ᐁ ᒥᔕᔨᑦ᙮ ᒪᒋᔕᑲᓄᐤ ᐧᐁᔥ ᐊᐧᐁᓐ ᐃᔅᑯᑕᒃ ᑳᐦ ᐊᔮᐧᐋᑦ ᐊᐧᐋᔑ ᓂᔮᓈᓄᐅᔑᑉ ᐁᒌ ᐃᑕᐦᑐᐳᓇᐧᐁᓯᑦ ᐅᔅᑳᒡ ᑳ ᐅᑕᐧᐋᔑᒥᑦ ᒉᒃ ᐁ ᐊᑎ ᓄᐧᐃᔨᒡ ᒉᒃ ᒫᒃ ᒦᒋᒻ ᐊᑖᐧᐋᐅᑲᒥᑯᐦᒡ ᐁ ᐋᐸᑎᓯᔨᓐ ᒉᒌ ᐅᐦᒋ ᑎᐸᐦᐊᒪᓐ ᒋᒪᓯᓇᐦᐄᑲᓐᐦ ᒥᓯᐧᐁ ᒫᒃ ᐧᐋᔥᑳ ᐁ ᐃᐦᑖᔨᓐ ᐁ ᐃᐦᑕᑯᐦᒡ ᒦᒋᒻ ᐁ ᒌᔕᑕᐦᒡ ᐁ ᒦᒋᔨᓐ ᒫᒃ ᐧᐁᔅ ᒋᑕᔦᔅᑯᔫᓐ ᐁ ᐸᐹᓈᔅᐱᓂᑕᐧᑖᐤ ᒋᑕᐧᐋᔒᒥᒡ ᐁ ᓂᑐᐧᐁᔨᐦᑕᒪᓐ ᒉᐧᑳᓐ ᒉᒌ ᐅᐦᒋ ᒥᔅᑰᒪᐦᒋᐦᐅᔨᓐ ᒋᔑᓄ ᒉᒌ ᓈᔅᐱᓂᑕᐧᑖᐤ᙮ 300 ᑎᐹᐯᑲᐦᐄᑲᓐ ᒌ ᐃᔅᐱᐦᑎᓂᑯᑑ, ᑖᐧᐯ ᑮᐸ ᒌ ᒥᔅᑕ ᒥᓯᒋᔥᑑ᙮ ᐋᐧᐁᔮ, ᓇᒧᐃ ᒣᒋᒻ ᐅᐦᒌ ᐴᔕ

« Je suis désolé, madame, dit doucement l'opérateur. Les règles de sécurité ne nous permettent pas de vous emmener sur ce manège. Cependant si vous marchez vers là-haut, indiqua-t-il en désignant où le manège s'achevait, vous pourrez retrouver votre famille quand ils descendront ».

Il était poli et parlait doucement.

Jennifer fit un signe de tête, descendit de l'enclos et se dirigea vers l'endroit où elle retrouverait sa famille. Elle voulait disparaître.

Bien sûr, elle avait du mal à bouger son corps – le simple fait de regarder une colline et de penser à la grimper la faisait pleurer. Bien sûr, elle était grosse – elle plaisantait sur son cul d'arbre de Noël plus fort que n'importe qui dans la pièce. Un gros cul, c'est ce qui arrive quand on commence à avoir des enfants à 18 ans et qu'on continue à en avoir jusqu'à ce qu'Il y en ait quatre, puis qu'on trouve un emploi dans une épicerie pour aider à payer les factures et qu'on est constamment entouré de malbouffe, et qu'on en mange parce qu'on est tellement épuisé de courir après ses enfants et qu'il faut de l'énergie pour continuer à leur courir après. Ok, ok, elle pesait 300 livres et c'était vraiment

"I'm sorry ma'am," the ride operator said gently. "The safety regulations won't allow us to take you on this ride. But if you walk up there," and he pointed to where the ride ended, "you can meet your family when they step off."

He was polite and spoke softly.

Jennifer nodded, stepped down from the enclosure, and headed up to where she would meet her family. She wanted to disappear.

Sure, she had a hard time moving her body – just looking at a hill and thinking about walking up would make her cry. Sure, she was a big girl – she joked about her Christmas tree ass louder than anyone in the room. A big ass is what happens when you start having kids at 18 and keep on having them until there are four of 'em, and then you get a job at a grocery store to help pay the bills and you're surrounded by junk food all the time, and you eat it because you're so friggin' exhausted from chasing after your kids and you need energy to keep chasing after them. Okay okay, she was 300 lbs and that was really big. But too big for an amusement park ride? She really wished

ᒋᔅᒑᔨᐦᑎᒻ ᓈᔥᒡ ᐋᐦ ᒥᓯᒋᔅᑎᒃ᙮ ᐧᐋᐧᐋᒡ ᐋ̈ᑲ ᒌᐦ ᒫᑯᐱᒌᓯᑦ ᐋᐦ ᐧᐄᐦ ᐴᓯᑦ ᐊᓂᑖᐦ ᐋᐦ ᒫᑎᐧᐋᓂᐧᐃᐧᐃᔭᒡ᙮ ᑭᒫ ᐋ̈ᑲ ᐅᐦᒋ ᐧᐋᐱᑎᐦᒡ ᐅᔮ ᓂᑎᐧᐋᔑᔒᒥᒡ, ᐄᑖᔨᐦᑎᒻ᙮

ᐊᓂᔮ ᒫᒃ ᑳ ᐹᒋ ᒌᐧᐋᒡ ᐊᓂᑖᐦ ᐅᐦᒋ ᒥᓅᓐᓛᓐ ᐊᓂᑎᐦ ᓈᔥᒡ ᑳ ᒦᒑᔨᐦᑖᑯᓂᔨᒡ ᐊᓂᔮ ᐋᐦ ᒌᐦ ᐧᐄᐦ ᐊᔨᐧᐋᔑᒡ ᑭᔮᐦ ᐧᐄᐦ ᒧᒋᑭᐦᑖᒡ, ᐋᑯᑎᐦ ᑳ ᒋᔅᒑᔨᐦᑎᐦᒃ ᐊᓂᔮᐦ ᑳ ᒥᐧᔮᐹᐅᔑᔨᒡᐦ ᐅᐧᐹᔨᒻᐦ ᑭᔮᐦ ᓈᐤ ᐊᓂᔮᐦ ᐅᑎᐧᐋᔑᔑᒻᐦ ᐅᐦᑖᐧᐄᔨᐤᐦ ᒑ ᓂᑭᑎᑯᑦ᙮ ᑭᔮᐦ ᐋᑯᑎᐦ ᑳ ᒋᔅᒑᔨᐦᑎᐦᒃ = ᐊᓂᔮᐦ ᑳ ᐄᑎᑯᑦ ᑯᑎᒃᐦ ᐊᐧᐋᔨᐤᐦ ᐋᐦ ᒌᐦ ᐧᐄᒑᐧᐋᑦ = ᔖᔥ ᐊᓂᑖᐦ ᐹᔨᑯᐱᐳᓐᐦ ᑯᑎᒃᐦ ᐃᔅᐧᑳᐤᐦ ᐋᐦ ᒌᐦ ᐧᐄᒑᐧᐋᔨᑯᐱᓈᓂᐦᐄ᙮ ᐊᓂᔮ ᒫᒃ ᑳ ᐄᔥᐱᔑ ᐃᐦᑖᒡ ᐊᓂᑖᐦ ᒥᓅᓐᓛᓐ ᑳᐦ ᐄᑖᑯᐱᓈ ᐊᓂᔮᐦ ᐅᒋᔥᐧᑳᔑᔒᒻᐦ ᔖᔥ ᐋᐦ ᒌᐦ ᓂᑭᑖᑦ ᒉᓂᕃᑫᐦ ᑭᔮᐦ ᐊᓂᔮᐦ ᐊᐧᐋᔑᔥᐦ᙮ ᑭᔮᐦ ᒫᒃ ᐊᓂᔮ, ᒨᔥ ᐋᐦ ᒌᐦ ᐃᔨᑦ ᐋ̈ᑲ ᐊᑎᑎᐤ ᐧᐄᐦ ᐃᔮᐧᐋᑦ ᒦᓐ ᐊᐧᐋᔑᔥᐦ ᔖᔥ ᐋᐦ ᒌᐦ ᐅᑯᔑᐦᐋᑯᐱᓈ ᐊᓂᔮᐦ ᐅᒋᔥᐧᑳᔑᔒᒻᐦ᙮ ᐊᓂᔮ ᒫᒃ ᒑᐧᑳᔨᐤ ᒫᐅᒡ ᐋ̈ᑲ ᐅᐦᒋ ᒥᔦᐧᐃᓈᑯᓃᒡ ᐋᔦᐧᐃᒄ ᐊᓂᔮᐦ ᐋᐦ ᒌᐦ ᐧᐄᒋᐦᐄᑯᑦ ᐊᓂᔮᐦ ᐅᑖᓂᓯᐧᐋᐤᐦ ᐋᐦ ᑳᑐᐧᐋᒡ ᒉᓂᕃᑫᐦ ᐊᓂᔮ ᑳ ᐅᒋᔥᐧᑳᔑᔒᒥᑯᐱᓈ᙮

ᐊᓂᔮᐦ ᑳ ᒥᐧᔮᐹᐅᔑᔨᒡᐦ ᑭᔮᐦ ᑳ ᐱᐱᒋᔅᑭᓈᐱᔨᒡᐦ ᐅᐹᔨᒻᐦ ᓈᔥᒡ ᐋ̈ᑲ ᑯᐃᔅᒄ ᐅᐦᒋ ᐃᐦᑐᑖᑯᑦ᙮

ᓂᐧᐃᒡ ᒫᒃ ᒥᔥᑏᐦ ᒌᐦ ᐃᐦᑎᑯᓂᔨᐤ ᒑᐧᑳᔨᐤ ᒑ ᒫᒥᑐᓈᔨᐦᑎᒥᐦᐄᑯᑦ᙮

ᑳᐸᐹ̈ᒫᐱᐦᒉᐸᔨᔨᒡ ᐧᐁᓰ ᐁ ᒥᓯᒋᔥᑎᑦ᙮ ᑲᒫ ᐁᑳ ᐅᐦᒋ ᐃᐦᑖᐧᐋᑯᓇᓀᓂᒡ ᐊᓂᑕ ᓂᑕᐧᐋᔒᒥᒡ ᒌ ᐃᑌᔨᐦᑕᒻ᙮

ᐃᔅᑯᑕᒃ ᒫᒃ ᑳᐧᐁᐸᔨᔨᐧᑖᐤ ᑳᒌᔑ ᐸᐹᒥᐸᔨᐧᑖᐤ ᐊᓂᑌ ᒪᓅᓐᓛᓐᑦ ᑳ ᐃᔅᐸᔨᐧᑖᐤ, ᐁᒄ ᑳ ᓇᑲᑎᑯᑦ ᐅᐧᐄᐦᑵᔮᓐ ᐅᐦᑖᐧᐋᐤᐦ ᐊᓂᔦᐦ ᑳ ᓀᐧᐃᔨᒡ ᐅᐧᑖᔒᒻᐦ᙮ ᒉᒃ ᐹᑎᒫ ᑳ ᒋᔅᒉᔨᐦᑕᐦᒃ ᐊᓂᔦᐦ ᐅᐧᐄᐦᑵᔮᒻ = ᐊᓂᔦ ᑳ ᐃᑎᑯᑦ ᐁ ᐧᐄᐦᑵᔮᒥᑦ ᐧᐄ = ᒌ ᐊᔮᐧᐁᔦᐦ ᐃᔅᑵᐤ ᓵᔅ ᐯᔭᒄ ᐱᐳᓐᐦ ᐁᒌ ᐧᐄᒉᐧᐋᑯᐸᓀᓐ᙮ ᒉᐧᑳᒡ ᐊᓂᑌ ᒪᓅᓐᓛᓐᑦ ᑳ ᐃᐦᑖᐧᑖᐤ ᒌ ᐃᑌᑯᐸᓀ ᐊᓂᔦᐦ ᐃᔅᑵᐤᐦ ᓵᔅ ᐁᒌ ᓇᑲᑖᑦ ᒉᓂᕃᑫᐦ ᓀᔅᑕ ᐅᑕᐧᐋᔒᒧᐧᐋᐤᐦ᙮ ᑲᔦ ᒫᒃ, ᐋᑦ ᐁᒌ ᐃᐧᑌᑯᐸᓀ ᐁᑳ ᒦᓐ ᐁ ᓂᑐᐧᐁᔨᒫᑦ ᐊᐧᐋᔕ, ᒌ ᐅᑕᐧᐋᔑᒥᐦᐁᑯᐸᓀ ᐊᓂᔦ ᐅᑕᒃ ᒃᐃᔅᑵᐤ᙮ ᓈᔅᒡ ᒫᒃ ᐁᒌᐧᐄ ᐃᐦᑎᑦ ᑲᔦ ᐁᒌ ᐄᑯᐸᓀᑦ ᐊᓂᔦᐦ ᐅᑖᓂᔕ ᐁᑳ ᒉᒌ ᐧᐄᐦᑕᒧᐧᐋᔨᒡ ᐅᑳᐧᐄ ᑯᑕᒃ ᐃᔅᑵᐤ ᐁ ᐧᐄᒉᐧᐋᑦ᙮

ᑖᐧᐯ ᐧᐄ ᐃᐦᑑ ᒌ ᐃᑌᔨᒣᐤ ᐊᓂᔦᐦ ᐅᐧᐄᐦᑵᔮᒻ ᑳ ᐧᐋᓴᑲᒥᑐᐧᐋᐱᔨᒡ ᐁ ᒥᐧᔮᐯᐅᑦ ᑳ ᐃᑌᔨᒫᑦ᙮

ᓈᔅᒡ ᑖᐧᐯ ᒌ ᐋᔨᒥᐦᐄᑰ ᐅᔦ᙮

beaucoup. Mais trop grosse pour un manège dans parc d'attraction ? Elle aurait vraiment aimé que ses enfants ne voient pas ça.

her kids hadn't seen that.

Quand ils rentrèrent de l'enfer de leurs vacances à Marineland, elle découvrit que son beau chum et le père de ses quatre enfants la quittait. Et puis, elle découvrit que lui, qui l'avait accusée de le tromper, voyait une autre femme depuis un an déjà. Que pendant toute la durée des vacances familiales à Marineland, il avait dit à sa blonde qu'il avait déjà quitté Jennifer et les enfants. Et que lui, qui avait toujours dit qu'il ne voulait pas d'autres enfants, avait mis cette autre fille enceinte. Et, pire encore, qu'il avait fait mentir leur fille à Jennifer pour l'aider à dissimuler sa liaison.

When they got home from their Marineland vacation from hell, she found out her handsome boyfriend and father of her four kids was leaving her. And then she found out that he – who had accused her of cheating – had been seeing another woman for a year already. That through the whole family vacation at Marineland he had been telling his girlfriend he had already left Jennifer and the kids. And that he, who had always said he didn't want more kids, had gotten that other girl pregnant. And, worst of all, that he had made their daughter lie to Jennifer to help cover up his affair.

Son beau *chum* aux yeux bleus était, en fait, un trou du cul.

Her handsome blue-eyed boyfriend was kind of an asshole.

Ça faisait beaucoup à encaisser.

It was a lot to take in.

ᑖᐧᐹᐦ ᒫᒃ ᓈᔥᑖᐧᐹᐦ ᒥᔥᑏᐦ ᒌᐦ ᐃᐦᑎᑯᓂᔨᐤ ᑫᓂᕕᕐ ᒑᐧᑳᔨᐤ ᒑ ᒥᑯᔅᑳᑖᔨᐦᑎᒥᐦᐄᑯᑦ ᑭᔮᐦ ᓈᔥᒡ ᐋᑳ ᐅᐦᒋ ᒥᔪᑐᑖᑯᑦ᙮

ᐧᐋᐦ ᐅᑎᓂᐦᒃ ᐊᓂᔮ ᒑᐧᑳᔨᐤ ᒑ ᓂᐦᐄᐧᐋᐦᐄᑯᑦ = ᒥᒄ ᒫᒃ ᒌᐦ ᒋᐱᐦᒋᐦᐄᓰ᙮ ᓂᒥᔮᔨᐤ ᐊᓂᔮ ᒑᐧᑳᔨᐤ ᒑ ᒦᒋᑦ ᓈᑎᐧᐋᔨᐦᑎᐦᒃ᙮ ᐊᓂᑖᐦ ᑭᐱᑎᐦᒡ ᐋᑐᐦᑖᑦ ᑭᔮᐦ ᐋᔫᐧᐃᒄ ᐧᐋᑎᓂᐦᒃ ᐊᓂᔮ ᑳ ᒥᔥᑭᐧᐋᑭᒥᔨᒡ, ᒥᒄ ᒫᒃ ᓂᒥᔮᔨᐤ ᑭᔮᐦ ᐊᓂᔮ ᓈᔥᒡ ᓈᑎᐧᐋᔨᐦᑎᐦᒃ᙮ ᓂᒧᐃ ᑳᑭᔮᐦ ᑯᑫᐃᓂᔨᐤ᙮ ᐧᐋᑎᓂᐦᒃ ᐊᓂᔮ ᒑ ᒌᐦ ᐅᐦᒋ ᐊᔨᒥᐦᐋᑦ ᐊᓂᔮᐦ ᑳ ᒌ ᐅᐦᑎᓂᒫᑯᑦ ᒥᒄ ᒫᒃ ᒦᓐ ᒌᐦ ᐱᒋᔅᑎᓂᒻ᙮ ᓂᒥᔮᔨᐤ ᑭᔮᐦ ᑯᑫᐃᓂᔨᐤ ᓈᑎᐧᐋᔨᐦᑎᐦᒃ᙮

ᐊᓂᔮ ᒫᒃ ᒑᐧᑳᔨᐤ ᑳ ᓂᑎᐧᐋᔨᐦᑎᐦᒃ, ᐊᓂᔮ ᒑᐧᑳᔨᐤ ᓈᔥᒡ ᑳ ᓂᑎᐧᐋᔨᐦᑎᐦᒃ, ᐋᔫᐧᐃᒄ ᒥᒄ ᐋᐦ ᐧᐄᐦ ᐱᐹᒧᐦᑖᑦ᙮ ᓈᔥᒡ ᐋᐦ ᒌᐦ ᑯᔥᐧᑳᔨᐦᑎᐦᒃ ᐅᔮ ᐋᐦ ᐧᐄᐦᑎᒃ ᐊᓂᔮ ᑭᔨᐧᐹ ᑯᑎᒃᐦ ᐊᐧᐋᔨᐤᐦ ᐋᐦ ᒌᐦ ᐧᐄᒑᐧᐋᔨᒡᐦ ᐊᓂᔮᐦ ᐅᐧᐹᔨᒻᐦ᙮

ᑳᐦ ᔮᔥᒋᔥᑭᐦᒃ ᑫᓂᕕᕐ ᐊᓂᔮᐦ ᒫᐅᒡ ᑳ ᒥᔫᔥᑭᐦᒃ ᐅᒥᔅᒋᓯᓐᐦ ᑭᔮᐦ ᓈᑖᐦ ᐋᑐᐦᑖᑦ ᐋᐦ ᐧᐋᔅᑳᐦᑖᓂᐧᐃᐧᐃᔨᒡ ᑭᔮᐦ ᑳᐦ ᐋᑎ ᐧᐋᔅᑳᐦᑖᑦ᙮ ᑭᔨᐧᐹ ᑳ ᒥᓯᒋᔅᑎᒃ ᑭᔮᐦ ᓂᒧᐃ ᐅᐦᒋ ᐄᔨᔥᐱᔑ ᐧᐋᐦᒌᐤ ᐋᐦ ᐱᐹᒧᐦᑖᑦ ᑳ ᐃᐦᑎᔨᒡᐦ ᐊᓂᔮᐦ ᐅᑎᐧᐋᔑᔒᒻᐦ᙮ ᓈᔥᒡ ᐋᐦ ᒌᐦ ᓂᓈᐦᑲᒋᔨᑯᑦ ᐊᓂᔮ ᐋᐦ ᐧᐄᐦ ᐱᒧᐦᑖᑦ᙮ ᐹᔨᐧᑳᐤ ᒫᒃ ᑳ ᒌᔑ ᐧᐋᔅᑳᐦᑖᑦ, ᓈᔥᒡ ᐋᐦ ᒌᐦ ᒋᓯᓯᑦ᙮ ᓂᔮᐧᔭᐤ ᑳᐦ ᐧᐋᔅᑳᐦᑖᑦ, ᓈᔥᒡ ᐋᐦ ᒌᐦ ᐃᔮᔨᐧᐄᑦ᙮ ᒥᑖᐦᐧᑖᐤ

ᑖᐧᐯ ᒌ ᐋᐃᒪᓂᔫ ᑖᓐ ᑳ ᐃᔅᐸᔨᑦ ᐁᒄ ᓈᔅᒡ ᑳᐧᐄ ᒋᔅᑳᔦᔨᐦᑕᒥᐦᐄᑯᑦ᙮

ᒧᐧᐁᐦᒡ ᒌ ᐧᐄᐦ ᐅᑎᓇᒻ ᐧᒑᑲᓚᑎᔫ ᑫᒌ ᐅᐦᒋ ᒥᔦᐦᑕᒃ = ᐁᑯᔥ ᓇᒧᐃ ᑳ ᐃᑌᔨᐦᑕᐦᒃ᙮ ᓇᒪᔦᔫ ᐧᐄ ᒦᒋᒥᔫ ᑳ ᓂᑐᐧᐁᔨᐦᑕᐦᒃ᙮ ᑳ ᓈᑕᐦᒃ ᐅᑲᐸᑎᒻ ᑳᐧᐄ ᐅᑎᓇᐦᒃ ᐊᓂᔫ ᐃᔅᑯᑌᐧᐋᐴᔫ, ᒥᒄ ᒫᒃ ᓇᒪᔦᔫ ᔮᐸᒡ ᐊᓂᔫ ᔮᐸᒡ ᑳ ᓂᑐᐧᐁᔨᐦᑕᐦᒃ᙮ ᒪᒋᓂᑐᐦᑯᐃᓐ ᒫᒃ ᐧᐄ, ᒌ ᐃᑌᔨᐦᑕᒻ᙮ ᒨᔥ ᒌ ᒥᔫᒪᐦᒋᐦᐆ ᐁ ᐃᐦᑑᑕᐦᒃ ᐊᓂᔫ᙮ ᑳ ᐅᑎᓇᐦᒃ ᑖᐦᑳᐱᐦᑫᓂᑲᓂᔫ, ᑫ ᐊᔨᒥᐦᐋᑦ ᐊᓂᔫ ᐊᐧᐁᔫᐦ ᑳᒌ ᐊᑖᒥᑯᑦ ᐁᒄ ᐋᐦᒌᐤᐦ ᑳ ᐅᐦᒋ ᐃᑌᔨᐦᑕᐦᒃ, ᑳᐤ ᑳ ᐊᑯᑖᑦ ᐊᓂᔫ ᑖᐦᑳᐱᐦᑫᓂᑲᓂᔫ᙮ ᓇᒧᐃ ᐧᐄ ᐊᓐ ᑳ ᐧᐋᐹᒡ ᒪᒋᓂᑐᐦᑯᐃᓐ ᓂᑲ ᐅᐦᒋ ᐧᐄᒋᐦᐄᑯᓐ ᒌ ᐃᑌᔨᐦᑕᒻ᙮

ᐊᓂᔫ ᑫᐧᑳᔫ ᑫ ᐧᐄᒋᐦᐄᑯᑦ, ᒋᐦᒋᐧᐁ ᑫ ᐧᐄᒋᐦᐄᑯᑦ, ᐁᐅᒄ ᑫᒌ ᓂᑑ ᐱᒧᐦᑌᑦ᙮ ᒌ ᑯᔥᐧᑫᔨᐦᑕᒥᐦᐄᑰ ᐅᔫ ᐁ ᐃᑌᔨᐦᑕᐦᒃ ᒧᐧᐁᐦᒡ ᑳ ᐃᔥᐱᔥ ᑯᔥᑯᐸᔨᑦ ᑳ ᐧᐄᐦᑕᒫᑯᑦ ᐅᐧᐄᐦᐧᑫᔮᒻ ᐁ ᓇᑲᑎᑯᑦ᙮

ᑳ ᒫᐦᑯᐱᑕᐦᒃ ᐊᓂᔫ ᒫᐅᒡ ᑳ ᒥᔦᐦᑕᐦᒃ ᐅᒪᔅᒋᓯᓐᐦ ᐁᒄ ᑳ ᓂᑑ ᐱᒧᐦᑌᑦ ᓀᑌ ᑳᒌ ᑲᒌᓂᐧᑳᓂᐦᑖᓄᔨᒡ᙮ ᒌ ᒥᓯᒋᔥᑑ ᓇᒧᐃ ᐅᐦᒌ ᐃᔥᐱᔥ ᒥᔫᐱᒧᐦᑌᐤ ᒧᐧᐁᐦᒡ ᐅᑕᐧᐋᔒᒻᐦ ᐁ ᐃᔥᐱᔥ ᐧᐁᐦᒋᐦᐄᑯᔨᒡ᙮ ᒌ ᐅᐦᐱᒣᐸᔨᐦᐆ ᐁᐧᐄ ᐅᑕᐦᐊᒣᑦ ᐁᑯᓐ ᐱᔑᒄ ᑳ ᐃᔑᓈᑯᓯᑦ᙮ ᐯᔨᐧᑳᐤ ᒌ ᒌᓂᐦᐧᑲᓂᐦᑌᐤ ᓄᐧᐋᒡ ᒫᒃ ᒌ ᐊᐳᐧᐁᐧᐄᐤ᙮ ᐃᔅᑯᑕᒃ ᓂᔮᔨᐧᓈᐤ ᑳ ᒌᓂᐧᑳᓂᐦᑌᑦ ᒥᒍᓐ ᒌ ᐃᔅᐱᔩᐤ᙮ ᔮᐸᒡ ᒫᒃ, ᐃᔅᑯᑕᒃ ᒥᑖᐦᐧᑖᐤ ᑳ

Ça faisait *beaucoup* à encaisser et on peut dire que ça affecta beaucoup Jennifer.

It was *a lot* to take in and it kind of got under Jennifer's skin.

Elle tendit la main vers un réconfort en forme de barre de chocolat et s'arrêta. Elle n'avait envie pas vraiment envie de nourriture. Elle alla dans son armoire de cuisine et tendit la main vers la bouteille de vodka à la place, mais elle n'en n'avait pas vraiment envie non plus. Peut-être un peu de cocaïne ? Ça lui permettait toujours de sentir très bien. Elle prit le téléphone pour appeler son dealer et reposa le combiné sur sa base. Elle n'avait pas non plus envie de cocaïne.

She reached for some chocolate-bar comfort – and stopped. Food wasn't really what she wanted. She went to her cupboard and reached instead for the vodka bottle, but she didn't really want that either. Maybe some blow? That always made her feel amazing. She picked up the phone to call her dealer and set it back down on the cradle. Cocaine wasn't it either.

Ce dont elle avait envie, ce dont elle avait vraiment, vraiment envie, c'était de sortir prendre une marche. Et il s'agissait là d'une surprise aussi grande que le fait que son chum la trompait.

What she wanted, what she really really wanted, was to go for a walk. And that was as big a surprise as her boyfriend cheating on her.

Jennifer attacha ses chaussures les plus confortables et marcha jusqu'à la piste où elle commença à faire le tour. Elle était grosse et elle ne pouvait pas marcher sans effort comme ses enfants le faisaient. Elle devait déplacer son poids d'un côté et balancer sa jambe vers l'avant pour faire un pas, puis déplacer son poids de l'autre côté pour faire le

Jennifer tied on her most comfortable shoes and walked to the track and began to go around. She was a big girl and she couldn't walk effortlessly like her kids did. She had to shift her weight to the one side, swing her leg around to take a step, and then shift it to the other side for the next step. By the end of the first lap, she was sweating. By the end of the fifth lap,

ᑳᐦ ᐧᐋᔅᑳᐦᑖᑦ, ᒑᑳᑦ ᓂᒥ ᐅᐦᒋ ᒌᐦ ᐋᐦᒌᐤ᙮ ᐊᔮᐱᒡ ᒫᒃ, ᐊᔮᐱᒡ ᒌᐦ ᐧᐋᔅᑳᐦᑖᐤ ᓃᔥᑎᓂᐤ ᑎᐦᐧᑖᐤ ᑳᐦ ᐅᑎᐦᒋᐱᔨᐦᑖᑦ ᐋᐦ ᐧᐋᔅᑳᐦᑖᑦ᙮

ᒦᓐ ᐊᓂᔮ ᐧᐃᔮᐱᓂᔨᒡ, ᒦᓐ ᐊᔮᐱᒡ ᑳ ᐃᐦᑐᑎᐦᒃ᙮

ᒋᒋᔅᒑᔨᐦᑖᓐ ᐋ, ᐄᑖᔨᐦᑎᒻ ᐊᓂᔮ ᒫᐧᑳᒡ ᐋᐦ ᐱᒧᐦᑖᑦ, ᐆ ᐋᐦ ᐱᒧᐦᑖᓂᐧᐃᒡ, ᓂᐧᐃᒡ ᐋᔨᒥᓐ᙮ ᐊᑎᑎᐤ ᒫᒃ ᓂᑭ ᐃᐦᑐᑖᓐ᙮ ᓃᔥᑎᓂᐤ ᑎᐦᐧᑖᐤ ᓂᑭ ᐧᐋᔅᑳᐦᑖᓐ ᐹᔨᑯᒌᔑᑳᐤᐦ, ᐋᔑᑯᒥᒌᔑᑳᐤᐦ, ᐹᔨᑯᐲᓯᒻ᙮ ᐋᑯᐦ ᐄᔮᑯ ᒑ ᐴᓂᔮᓐ᙮

ᒫᐧᑳᒡ ᒫᒃ ᐊᓂᔮ ᐋᐦ ᐱᐧᐹᒧᐦᑖᑦ, ᒌᐦ ᒋᔅᒋᓰᑎᑎᐧᐋᐤ ᐊᓂᔮᐦ ᐅᐧᐹᔨᒻᐦ᙮ ᐄᐦᐄ, ᓈᔥᑖᐧᐹᐦ ᒌᐦ ᐱᐱᒋᔅᑭᓈᐱᔨᐤᐦ ᑭᔮᐦ ᒥᐦᒑᑐ ᐃᔅᐧᑳᐤᐦ ᒌᐦ ᒧᔥᑖᓈᑯᔨᐤᐦ, ᒥᑯ ᒫᒃ ᑖᐹ ᐋᐱᑎᓂᔨᐤ ᒥᑯ ᐋᐦ ᒥᐧᔮᐹᐅᔑᑦ ᐊᐧᐋᓐ᙮ ᐊᓂᔮ ᒫᒃ ᐋᑳ ᔔᔥ ᐃᐦᑖᔨᐤᐦ ᐊᓂᑎᐦ ᐋᐦ ᐄᐦᑖᒡ, ᒑᒃ ᓂᒥ ᐅᐦᒋ ᒋᔅᒋᓰᑎᑎᐧᒫᐤ ᐊᓂᔮᐦ ᐋᐦ ᐱᐱᒋᔅᑭᓈᐱᔨᒡᐦ, ᑭᔮᐦ ᓂᒧᐃ ᐅᐦᒋ ᒥᐦᑖᑎᐧᒫᐤ ᐊᓂᔮ ᓂᔮᓂᑯᑑᓐᐦ ᐋᐦ ᒌᐦ ᒫᒫᐦᒋᔨᑎᑯᑦ ᐋᐦ ᐄᑎᑯᑦ ᐋᐦ ᐧᐋᔦᒻ ᑖᐦᒋᐳᑦ ᑭᔮᐦ ᐋᐦ ᒥᒋᓯᑦ᙮ ᐊᑎᑎᐤ ᒌᐦ ᒥᔫᐦᑖᑯᓃᔨᐤ ᐊᓂᑖᐦ ᐧᐄᒋᐦᐧᐋᐦᒡ ᐋᑳ ᐹᐦᑖᑯᓯᔨᒡᐦ ᐊᓂᔮ ᐋᐦ ᐄᑎᑯᑦ᙮ ᒑᒃ ᓈᔥᑎᔨᒡ ᓂᒥ ᐅᐦᒋ ᒥᐦᑖᑖᐤ᙮ ᒥᑯ ᒫᒃ ᒋᑭ ᓂᑎᐧᐋᔨᒫᐤ ᒉᓂᕕᕐ ᔓᐧᐄᔮᓐᐦ ᑳ ᒌᐦ ᐅᐦᒋ ᐱᒥᓈᑦ ᐅᑎᐧᐋᔑᔒᒻᐦ = ᐧᐄᒋᐦᐄᐧᐋᐅᒦᒋᒥᔨᐤ ᒋᑭ ᓂᑎᐧᐋᔨᐦᑎᒧᒡ ᐹᑎᔥ ᒌᐦ ᒥᔅᑭᐦᑳ

ᒌᓂᐧᑳᓂᐦᑌᑦ ᓂᑲ ᓂᐱᓐ ᒌ ᐃᑌᔨᐦᑕᒻ᙮ ᔮᐸᒡ ᒫᒃ ᒦᓐ ᒌ ᐱᒧᐦᑌᐤ, ᓇᒧᐃ ᐅᐦᒋ ᐴᓃᐤ ᐹᑎᔅ ᓃᔥᑐᓀᐧᐋᐤ ᑳ ᒌᓂᐧᑳᓂᐦᑌᑦ᙮

ᒦᓐ ᑳ ᒌᔑᑳᔨᒡ ᐁᑯ ᒦᓐ ᑳ ᐱᒧᐦᑌᑦ᙮

“ᒋ ᒋᔅᒉᔨᐦᑌᓐ ᐋ ᒉᐧᑳᓐ,” ᒌ ᐃᑎᓲ ᐊᓂᔫ ᐁ ᐱᒧᐦᑌᑦ, “ᓇᒧᐃ ᒥᒍᓐ ᒥᔦᔨᐦᑖᑯᓐ ᐁ ᐱᒧᐦᑖᓅᐦᒡ᙮ ᔮᐸᒡ ᒥᑯ ᓲᐦᒃ ᓂᑲ ᐱᒧᐦᑌᓐ᙮ ᓃᔥᑐᓀᐧᐋᐤ ᓂᑲ ᒌᓂᐧᑳᓂᐦᑌᓐ ᒉᔑᑯᒻ ᒌᔑᑳᐤ, ᐯᔮᑯ ᐲᓯᒻ ᐃᔥᐱᔥ᙮ ᐁᑯ ᒫᒃ ᒉ ᐴᓂᔮᓐ᙮”

ᐊᓂᔫ ᒫᒃ ᐁ ᐱᒧᐦᑌᑦ ᒌ ᒫᒥᑐᓀᔨᒣᐤ ᐅᐧᐄᐦᐧᑫᔮᒻ᙮ ᑖᐧᐯ ᑮᐹ ᐧᐋᔕᑲᒥᑐᐧᐋᐴ, ᒥᐧᔮᔑᔫᐦ ᐅᔅᒌᔑᑯᐦ ᒥᐦᒉᑐ ᐃᔅᐧᑫᐤ ᒌ ᓂᑐᐧᐁᔨᒥᑰ, ᒥᑯ ᒫᒃ ᓇᒧᐃ ᒉᐧᑳᓐ ᐋᑦ ᓈᔅᒡ ᐁ ᒥᐧᔮᐯᐅᑦ ᒌ ᐃᑌᔨᐦᑕᒻ᙮ ᔖᔅ ᓇᒧᐃ ᐅᐦᒋ ᐊᔮᐧᐁᐤ ᐊᓂᔫᐦ ᑳᐧᐋᔕᑲᒥᑐᐧᐋᐱᔨᒡ, ᔖᔅ ᓇᒧᐃ ᐅᐦᒋ ᐯᐦᑕᐧᐁᐤ ᐊᓂᔫ ᒨᔥ ᒉᒉᐦᐤ ᑳᒌ ᐃᑎᑯᑦ, ᒋ ᑖᐦᒋᐳᓐ ᑲᔪ ᒋ ᒪᒋᓯᓐ ᑳᒌ ᐄᑎᑯᑦ᙮ ᒌ ᒥᔦᔨᐦᑖᑯᓂᔫ ᐧᐄᒋᐦᒡ ᐁᑳ ᐯᐦᑖᑯᓯᔨᒡ ᐊᐧᐁᔫ ᐊᓂᔫ ᐁ ᐃᔑ ᐊᔨᒥᐦᐄᑯᑦ᙮ ᓇᒧᐃ ᐅᐦᒋ ᒥᐦᒉᑌᐤ ᒥᒍᓐ᙮ ᓇᒧᐃ ᑲᔦ ᒦᓐ ᒋᑲ ᐅᐦᒋ ᓅᐦᑌᐸᔫᒡ ᔔᓂᔮᔫ = ᐊᔓᒥᑯᓰᐧᐃᓂᔫ ᒋᑲ ᐱᒥᐸᔨᐦᐄᑰᒡ ᒉ ᐃᔥᐱᔥ ᐁᑳ ᒥᔅᑲᐦᒃ ᐋᐸᑎᓰᐧᐃᓂᔫ᙮ ᒌ ᐋᐃᒪᓂᔫ ᐊᓂᑕ ᒣᐧᑳᒡ᙮ ᒌ ᒫᑑ ᒫᓐᐦ ᐁ ᒫᒥᑐᓀᔨᐦᑕᐦᒃ ᐁ ᐃᔅᐸᔨᐧᑖᐤ᙮ ᒌ ᒫᑑ ᐁ ᒋᔅᒋᓯᑦ ᑕᐦᐧᑖᐤ ᑳ ᐋᐦᑯᐦᐄᑯᑦ ᐅᐧᐄᐦᐧᑫᔮᓐ᙮

pas suivant. À la fin du premier tour, elle transpirait. À la fin du cinquième tour, elle était épuisée. À la fin du dixième, elle était à moitié morte. Pourtant, elle continua à marcher jusqu'à ce qu'elle ait fait le tour de cette maudite piste vingt maudite fois.

Et le lendemain, elle recommença.

*Tu sais quoi, se disait-elle en marchant, ce truc de marcher, c'est plate. Je vais en faire plus. Vingt tours par jour, tous les jours, pendant un mois. Et puis j'arrêterai.*

Pendant qu'elle marchait, elle pensait à son chum. Bien sûr, il était Monsieur Les-yeux-bleus et beaucoup de femmes le voulaient, mais la beauté n'était pas tout. Maintenant qu'il était parti, ses yeux bleus étaient partis aussi, mais, c'est certain que tous les « grosse » et « moche » qu'il lui balançait de temps en temps ne lui manquaient pas. Les ondes sonores dans sa maison étaient bien plus heureuses sans tout ça. En fait, il ne lui manquait pas du tout. L'argent allait être un problème désormais – ses enfants et elle devraient se tourner vers l'aide sociale jusqu'à ce qu'elle trouve d'autres moyens de joindre les deux bouts. C'était

she was exhausted. By the end of the tenth, she was half dead. Still, she kept walking until she had gone around that friggin' track twenty friggin' times.

And the next day, she did it again.

*You know what,* she thought to herself as she walked, *this walking thing sucks. I'm gonna do more of it. Twenty laps a day, every day, for one month. And then I'll quit.*

While she walked, she thought about her boyfriend. Sure, he was Mr. Blue Eyes and a whole lot of women wanted him, but handsome isn't everything. Now that he was gone, his blue eyes were gone too, but she sure didn't miss hearing all that fat-and-ugly shit he hurled at her every now and then. The sound waves in her house were a whole lot happier without all that. She actually didn't miss him at all. Money was gonna be a problem now – she and her kids would have to go on welfare until she found other ways to make ends meet. That was stressful. Thinking about it made her cry. Remembering all the ways he had been mean to her made her cry.

ᐋᐱᑎᓰᐧᐃᓂᔨᐤ᙮ ᓈᔥᑖᐹᐦ ᒌᐦ ᒫᑯᔥᑳᑰ᙮ ᐊᓂᔮ ᐋᔑ ᒋᔅᒋᓯᒡᐦ ᑳ ᒌ ᒫᑐᑦ᙮ ᒑᔅᒌᑎᐧᐋᒡᐦ ᐊᓂᔮ ᑳ ᐄᔥᐱᔑ ᒥᒫᔮᔨᒥᑯᑦ ᐋᑯᑎᐦ ᒦᓐ ᑳ ᒌ ᒫᑐᑦ᙮

ᐋᑦ ᑭᔨᐧᐹ ᒌᐦ ᒫᑐᑦ ᒫᓐᐦ ᓂᔮᓂᑯᒎᓐᐦ, ᓈᓈᓂᒌᒻ ᒌᐦ ᐧᐋᐦᒋᐱᔨᔨᐤ ᐋᐦ ᐱᐧᐹᒧᐦᑖᑦ ᑭᔮᐦ ᓈᓈᓂᒌᒻ ᒌᐦ ᒥᐧᔮᔨᐦᑎᒻ᙮ ᒑᒃ ᑳ ᒌ ᐱᒧᐦᑖᑦ ᐋᐦ ᐄᑐᐦᑖᑦ ᐊᓂᑖᐦ ᐋᐦ ᐋᐱᑎᓰᑦ, ᑭᔮᐦ ᒥᒄ ᐊᓂᑖᐦ ᐧᐋᐦ ᐄᑐᐦᑖᑦ ᐋᑳ ᓈᔥᒡ ᐧᐋᐦᔫᐧᐃᓈᑯᓂᔨᒡ ᑳ ᒌᐦ ᐱᒧᐦᑖᑦ, ᑭᔮᐦ ᓂᒥ ᐅᐦᒋ ᐱᒧᐦᑖᐤ ᐊᓂᑖᐦ ᐋᐦ ᐄᔑ ᐹᔕᓈᑯᓂᔨᒡ ᐀ ᐊᓂᑖᐦ ᐊᑎᑎᐤ ᐋᐦ ᔮᐅᓈᑯᓂᔨᒡ ᐋᑯᑖᐦ ᑳ ᒌ ᐱᒧᐦᑖᑦ᙮

ᑳ ᐄᔥᐧᑳᑯᒋᓂᔨᒡᐦ ᐊᓂᔮᐦ ᐲᓯᒻᐦ, ᑳᐦ ᐄᑖᔨᐦᑎᐦᒃ ᐋᑳ ᒑ ᐴᓃᑦ ᐋᐦ ᐱᐹᒧᐦᑖᑦ᙮ ᐋᑯᑎᐦ ᓈᔥᒡ ᑳᐦ ᒥᔪᐱᔨᔨᒡ ᐋᐦ ᒫᒥᑐᓈᔨᐦᑎᐦᒃ᙮ ᐊᑎᑎᐤ ᑯᐃᔅᒄ ᐋᐦ ᐄᔑ ᒫᒥᑐᓈᔨᐦᑎᐦᒃ᙮ ᒌᐦ ᒥᔪᒥᐦᒋᐦᐆ ᒫᒃ᙮

ᐊᓂᔮ ᒫᒃ ᐋᐦ ᐱᐹᒧᐦᑖᑦ ᑳᐦ ᔒᐅᑖᑦ ᒉᓂᕕᕝ, ᐋᑯᑎᐦ ᑳ ᒌ ᒋᔅᒋᓰᑎᑎᒃᐦ ᒑ ᒦᒋᑦ ᐊᓂᔮ ᒑᐧᑲᔮᐤ ᐋᑳ ᓈᔥᒡ ᐧᐄᒋᐦᐄᑯᑦ ᐅᔮᐦᒡ, ᐊᓂᔮ ᑭᔨᐧᐹ ᒨᔥ ᑳ ᒌ ᒦᒋᑦ᙮

ᐄᐦᐄ, ᑭᔨᐧᐹ ᑳ ᒋᔅᒋᓰᑎᑎᒃᐦ, ᒌᐦ ᒋᔅᒑᔨᐦᑎᒻ ᐧᐋᔅ ᒥᔥᒌᐦ ᐋᐦ ᒦᒋᑦ ᐊᓂᔮ ᒐ ᐄᔥᐱᔑ ᒦᒋᑯᐱᓈ᙮ ᐧᑳᐧᔖᓐ ᒫᒃ ᒋᑭ ᒌᐦ ᐄᔑᓈᑯᓂᔨᐤ ᒐ ᐋᒋᐧᐃᓂᐦᒃ, ᒑ ᐊᒋᐧᐃᓂᐦᒃ ᐋᔑᑯᒥᒌᔑᑳᐤᐦ᙮

ᒌ ᒫᑑ ᒫᓐ ᒥᒄ ᒫᒃ ᒌ ᐧᐄᒋᐦᐄᑰ ᐁ ᐱᒧᐦᑌᑦ ᑲᔦ ᓇᒧᐃ ᐅᐦᒋ ᐃᔥᐱᔥ ᐊᔦᔅᑯᐦᑌᐤ ᐧᐁᑖᒡ ᒌ ᒥᔫᐱᒧᐦᑌᐤ᙮ ᒉᒃ ᒣᔑᑯᒻ ᒌᔑᑳᐤᐦ ᒌ ᐱᒧᐦᑌᐤ ᐁ ᓂᑑ ᐋᐸᑎᓯᑦ ᒫᒃ ᐧᐃᔦᔅ ᐁ ᐃᑐᐦᑌᑦ ᐁᑳ ᐲᐦᒑᔨᒡ ᒨᔥ ᑲᔦ ᒣᔅᑲᓈᐦᒡ ᒌ ᐱᒧᐦᑌᐤ ᓇᒧᐃ ᐧᐄ ᐊᓂᑌ ᐁ ᐱᔅᒣᔑᒧᔨᒡ ᒣᔅᑲᓈᔫ ᐁ ᑕᐦᐧᑳᔨᒡ ᐀ ᐅᔥᑌ ᓃᔕᑌᐧᐋᐤ ᒣᒌ ᐅᑕᐦᐊᒣᔮᓐ ᒌ ᐃᑌᔨᐦᑕᒻ᙮

ᐃᔅᑯᑕᒃ ᒫᒃ ᐯᔭᒄ ᐲᓯᒻ ᑳ ᐃᔥᐱᔥ ᐱᒧᐦᑌᑦ ᒉᒃ ᒌ ᒥᔦᔩᐦᑕᒻ ᐁ ᐱᒧᐦᑌᑦ ᐁᑯᓐ ᒫᒃ ᒨᔥ ᒣ ᐃᐦᑎᔮᓐ ᒌ ᐃᑌᔨᐦᑕᒻ᙮ ᒌ ᐧᐄᒋᐦᐄᑰ ᒣᒌ ᒫᒥᑐᓀᔨᐦᑕᐦᒃ᙮ ᒌ ᐱᔦᑲᔅᒋᒫᒥᑐᓀᔨᐦᑕᒻ᙮ ᒌ ᒥᔫᒪᐦᒋᐦᐆ ᑲᔦ᙮

ᒌ ᒨᔑᐦᑖᐤ ᒫᒃ ᐁᐧᐄ ᓰᐧᐁᔨᐦᑦ ᐯᒧᐦᑌᒡ ᒫᓐᐦ, ᐁᒄ ᑳᒌ ᒋᔅᒋᓰᑐᑕᐦᒃ ᒦᒋᒥᔫ ᐁᑳ ᒦᒋᒥᔅᑳᒣᔨᒡ᙮

ᑖᐧᐯ ᐧᐁᓯᓐ, ᐁᑯᓐ ᑳ ᐃᔑᓈᑯᓯᑦ ᐁ ᒫᒥᑐᓀᔨᒥᓯᑦ ᑮᐹ, ᐧᐄᔭ ᐁᑎᑑ ᒥᔅᑕᐦᐄ ᐁᒌ ᒦᒋᓯᑦ ᐃᔥᐱᔥ ᑯᑕᑲᒡ ᐊᐧᐁᓂᒌ᙮ ᓈᓂᑑ ᒋᐹᒌ ᑯᒋᐦᑖᐤ ᐁᑳ ᒉᒌ ᐃᔥᐱᔥ ᒦᒋᓯᑦ, ᐧᐁᑖᒡ ᐊᐱᔒᔥ ᒉᒌ ᒦᒋᑦ ᒉᐧᑲᔫ ᒣᔑᑯᒻ ᒌᔑᑳᐤ᙮

stressant. Penser à ça la faisait pleurer. Se souvenir de toutes les façons dont il l'avait maltraitée, la faisait pleurer.

Ce qui était bien, c'est que même avec les pleurs, la marche devenait plus facile et elle craignait moins. Elle commença donc à marcher tous les jours également pour se rendre au travail et à chaque endroit à distance de marche, où elle devait se rendre, en évitant toujours les raccourcis; si un chemin coupait à travers un terrain, elle faisait le tour pour accumuler vingt pas de plus.

The good thing was that even with the crying, walking was getting easier and sucking less. So she started walking to work every day too, and anywhere she needed to go that was in walking distance, always avoiding shortcuts – if a path cut across a yard, she walked around to collect twenty extra steps.

À la fin du mois, elle pensa qu'elle aimerait peut-être continuer à marcher. Cela lui donnait le temps de réfléchir, éclaircissait ses pensées, lui faisait du bien.

By the end of the month, she thought she might like to keep walking. It gave her time to think. Cleared her head. Felt okay.

La marche donnait faim à Jennifer, alors, naturellement, elle commençait à penser à du *junkfood*.

Walking made Jennifer hungry, so, naturally, she started thinking about junk food.

Ok, quand elle y réfléchissait vraiment, elle devait admettre qu'elle en mangeait plus que la plupart des gens. Peut-être qu'elle pourrait en réduire la quantité, un peu moins chaque jour.

Okay, when she really thought about it, she had to admit she ate more of it than most people. Maybe she could cut back, a little less of it every day.

ᑮᔮᐦ ᐧᑳᐧᔖᓐ ᒋᑭ ᒌᐦ ᑯᒋᔥᑖᐤ ᐹᔨᑯᐲᓯᒪᐦ ᐋᑳ
ᓈᔥᑎᔨᒡ ᒦᒋᑦ =

ᐧᐋᓵ᙮

ᓂᒧᐃ ᒋᑭ ᐧᐋᐦᑎᓂᔨᐤ᙮ ᐹᔨᑯᐲᓯᒪᐦ ᐋᐦ
ᐱᐹᒧᐦᑖᑦ ᑮᔮᐦ ᐋᐦ ᒋᓯᓯᑦ ᐊᑎᑎᐤ ᒌᐦ
ᐧᐋᐦᑖᔨᐦᑎᒻ ᐄᔥᐱᔑᐧᐄ ᐹᔨᐧᑯᐲᓯᒪᐦ ᐋᑳ
ᓈᔥᑎᔨᒡ ᒦᒋᑦ ᐧᒑᑭᓚᑦᐦ ᑮᔮᐦ ᐋᔨᐦᑯᓈᔥᐦ ᑮᔮᐦ
ᒋᐸᔅ ᑮᔮᐦ ᑳᔒᐧᐋᑭᒥᔒᔨᒡ᙮

ᒥᑯ ᒫᒃ ᓲᐦᒃ ᒋᑭ ᑯᒋᔥᑖᐤ᙮

ᑖᐹ ᐅᐦᒋ ᐧᐋᐦᑎᓂᔨᐤ ᐊᓂᔮ ᐹᔨᑯᐲᓯᒪᐦ ᑳ
ᐱᐹᒧᐦᑖᑦ᙮ ᐊᓂᔮ ᓃᔥᑎᒻ ᐹᔨᒄ ᐲᓯᒪᐦ ᐋᑳ
ᓈᔥᑎᔨᒡ ᐅᐦᒋ ᒦᒋᑦ ᐊᓂᔮ ᒑᐧᑳᔨᐤ ᐋᑳ ᒑ
ᐧᐄᒋᐦᐄᑯᑦ ᐅᔮᐦᒡ ᓈᔥᑖᐧᐹ ᒌᐦ ᐋᔨᒥᓂᔨᐤ᙮
ᓂᓈᐦᑰ ᒌᐦ ᑯᒋᔥᑖᐤ ᒑᐧᑳᔨᐤ ᒑ ᐧᐄᒋᐦᐄᑯᑦ
ᐊᓂᔮ ᐹᔨᑯᐲᓯᒻ᙮ ᑳ ᒌᐦ ᐅᔑᐦᐋᑦ ᒥᔅᑯᒦᐦ
ᑮᔮᐦ ᑳ ᒌᐦ ᐱᐲᓯᐦᐧᐋᑦ ᐋᔫᐧᐃᑯᓐᐦ ᑳ ᒌᐦ
ᒥᓂᐦᐧᑳᑦ ᒨᔮᒻ ᐋᐦ ᒥᓂᐦᐧᑳᔮᓐ ᑳᔒᐧᐋᑭᒥᔑᒡ
ᑳ ᒌ ᐄᑖᔨᐦᑎᐦᐦᒃ, ᐋᑦ ᐋᑳ ᐅᐦᒋ ᒥᓂᐦᐧᑳᑦ
ᑳᔒᐧᐋᑭᒥᔑᔨᒡ᙮ ᒥᑯ ᒫᒃ, ᐊᓂᔮ ᐋᑳ ᐅᐦᒋ
ᐋᐱᒋᐦᑖᑦ ᔖᑳᔨᐤ, ᓈᔥᒡ ᑳ ᒌᐦ ᓈᓈᒥᐱᔨᑦ
ᐋᔑᑯᒥᒌᔑᑳᐤᐦ᙮ ᐊᓂᔮ ᒫᒃ ᓈᔥᒡ ᐋᐦ ᒌᐦ
ᐄᔅᐱᔨᔨᒡᐦ ᐅᑎᐦᒌ ᓂᒥ ᒌᔨᐧᐋ ᐅᐦᒋ ᒌᐦ
ᑎᐦᑯᓂᒻ ᒥᓯᓂᐦᐄᑭᓈᐦᑎᑯᔨᐤ ᑮᔮᐦ ᒫᒃ ᓂᒥ
ᐅᐦᒋ ᒌᐦ ᒥᓯᓂᐦᐄᒑᐱᔨᐦᑖᐤ᙮ ᐋᑯᑎᐦ ᒑᒃ ᑳ
ᒌ ᒥᓂᐦᐧᑳᑦ ᑳᔒᐧᐋᑭᒥᔑᔨᒡ᙮ ᑏᐧᐋᐦᒡ ᑳ ᒌ
ᒋᐱᐦᒋᐱᔨᔨᒡ ᐊᓂᔮᐦ ᐋᐦ ᓈᓈᒥᐱᔨᑦ᙮

ᒫᒃ ᒋᐹ ᑯᒋᐦᑖᐤ ᐯᔭᒄ ᐲᓯᒻ ᐁᑳ ᒦᒋᑦ ᐯᔭᒄ
ᑫᐧᑳᔫ =

ᐧᑫᓵ ᑖᐧᐯ ᒋᑲ ᐋᐃᒪᓐ, ᒌ ᐃᑌᔨᐦᑕᒻ᙮

ᓇᒧᐃ ᑮᐹ ᑲᑕ ᐅᐦᒋ ᐧᐁᐦᑕᓐ᙮ ᐁᑎᔫ ᒌ
ᐧᐁᐦᑕᓐ ᐯᔭᒄ ᐲᓯᒻ ᐱᔑᒄ ᐁᒌ ᐱᒧᐦᑌᔮᓐ ᐁᒌ
ᐊᐧᐯᐧᐄᔮᓐ ᑖᐧᐯ ᑲᑕ ᐋᐃᒪᓐ ᐁᑳ ᒌ ᒦᒋᔮᓂ
ᐧᒑᑲᓚᑦ ᑲᔦ ᐋᐃᐦᑯᓈᓵᒡ, ᑳᑲᔅᐱᑌᐧᑳᐤ ᐸᑌᑎᔅ
ᑲᔦ ᐁᑳ ᒌ ᒥᓂᐦᐧᑫᔮᓂ ᑳ ᓰᐧᐋᑲᒥᔑᒡ᙮

ᒥᑯ ᒫᒃ ᔮᐸᒡ ᓂᑲ ᑯᒋᐦᑖᓐ, ᒌ ᐃᑌᔨᐦᑕᒻ᙮

ᐊᓂᔫ ᐅᔅᑲᒡ ᐯᒧᐦᑌᑦ ᐯᔭᒄ ᐲᓯᒻ ᐃᔥᐱᔥ
ᑖᐧᐯ ᐋᐃᒪᓐ ᒌ ᐃᑌᔨᐦᑕᒻ᙮ ᐯᔭᒄ ᐲᓯᒻ ᐁᑳ
ᐅᐦᒋ ᒦᒋᑦ ᒥᒋᒥᔫ ᐁᑳ ᒥᔫᔅᑳᑫᔨᒡ ᑖᐧᐯ ᒌ
ᐋᔨᒥᐦᐄᑯ᙮ ᒌ ᓈᓂᑐᐧᐁᔨᐦᑕᒻ ᑖᓐ ᑫᒌ ᐃᐦᑎᑦ
ᐁᐧᐄ ᔖᐳᔥᑲᐦᒃ ᐅᔫ᙮ ᒌ ᒥᔅᑰᒋᐦᑖᐤ ᓂᐱᔫ ᐁᒄ
ᑳᒌ ᐱᒋᔥᑲᐦᐧᐋᑦ ᐊᓂᔫᐦ ᒪᔅᑯᒦ ᐁ ᐅᔑᐦᑕᒫᓯᑦ
ᑫᐧᑳᔫ ᐁ ᒥᓂᐦᐧᑫᑦ ᒧᐧᐁᒡ ᑳᓰᐧᐋᑲᒥᔑᒡ ᐁ
ᒥᓂᐦᐧᑫᔮᓐ ᑫᒌ ᐃᑌᔨᐦᑕᐦᒃ ᐋᑦ ᒫᒃ ᐁᑳ
ᐃᐦᑕᑯᓂᔨᒡ ᐊᓂᑕ ᑳᓰᐧᐋᑲᒥᔑᔨᒡ᙮ ᔮᐸᒡ ᒫᒃ,
ᐋᑦ ᐁᑳ ᐃᔥᐱᔥ ᒦᒋᑦ ᐁ ᔕᑳᐅᓂᔨᒡ ᑫᐧᑳᔫ,
ᒣᔑᑯᒻ ᒌᔥᐧᑳᐱᐦᑖᒌᔑᑳᐤᐦ ᒌ ᓇᓇᒥᐸᔫ᙮ ᓇᒧᐃ
ᒣᒋᒻ ᐅᐦᒌ ᑕᐦᑯᓅ ᒪᓯᓇᐦᐄᑲᓈᐦᑎᒄ ᒫᒃ ᑫᒌ
ᒪᓯᓇᐦᐄᑫᐸᔨᐦᑖᑦ ᑳ ᐃᔥᐱᔥ ᒌ ᓇᓇᒥᐸᔨᑦ᙮
ᐁᑯᑦ ᑳ ᒌ ᒥᓂᐦᐧᑫᑦ ᑳᓰᐧᐋᑲᒥᔑᔨᒡ ᑫᒌ
ᐃᔥᑌᐸᔨᔨᒡ ᐁ ᓇᓇᒥᐸᔨᑦ᙮ ᑏᐧᐁᐦᒡ ᒫᒃ ᒌ
ᒋᐱᐦᒋᐸᓂᔫ ᐁ ᓇᓇᒥᐸᔨᑦ᙮

Ou elle pourrait essayer de passer un mois sans...

Ohhh là là.

*Ça,* ça ne serait pas facile. Un mois de marche et de transpiration semblait beaucoup plus facile qu'un mois sans barres de chocolat, sans biscuits, sans chips et sans boissons gazeuses.

Mais elle allait devoir essayer.

Le premier mois de marche avait été un défi. Le premier mois sans malbouffe fut sacrément brutal. Elle commença à inventer des trucs pour passer le mois. Elle congela de l'eau et pilla la glace pour en faire un slurpee, afin de pouvoir prétendre qu'elle buvait des boissons gazeuses, même si elle n'avait pas de boissons gazeuses chez elle. Toutefois, sans tout ce sucre auquel elle s'était habituée, elle était victime de tremblements tous les après-midis. Elle tremblait tellement qu'elle ne pouvait calmer suffisamment ses mains pour tenir un stylo ou taper sur un clavier. Elle devait alors être moins sévère avec elle-même et prendre un Pepsi. Immédiatement, les tremblements s'atténuaient.

Or she could try one month without it –

Ohhh man.

*That* was not gonna be easy. One month of walking and sweating seemed a whole lot easier than one month without chocolate bars and cookies and chips and pop.

But she was gonna have to try.

The first month of walking had been a challenge. The first month of no junk food was friggin' brutal. She started inventing tricks to get through the month. She froze water and crushed the ice into a slurpee so that she could still go through the motions of drinking pop, even if there was no pop there. But, without all the sugar she was used to, she got the shakes every afternoon. She would shake so badly that she couldn't still her hands enough to hold a pen or type. She had to ease up on herself then and have a Pepsi. Immediately the shakes would subside.

ᐋᔪᐧᐃᒄ ᐋᐦᑎᒃ ᐅᔮ ᐊᐧᐋᓐ ᓈᔥᒡ ᓈᐅᔥ ᐋᐦ ᒌᐦ ᐋᐱᒋᔥᑖᑦ ᒑᐧᑳᔮᐤ, ᒋᔥᒋᑯᒡ ᒫᒃ ᐋᐦ ᐴᓂᐦᑖᑦ᙮ ᐋᑯᑖᐦ ᐋᐦᑎᒡ ᐊᓂᒌ ᐧᐋᓂᒌ ᒥᒋᓂᑐᐦᑯᔮᓐᐦ ᐋᐦ ᐋᐱᒋᐦᑖᒡ᙮ ᓂᔮᓂᑯᑑᓐᐦ ᐧᐋᐧᐄᓵᐧᐋ ᐹᔮᑯᑎᐧᐃᔥᑖᐤᐦ ᐱᒦᐦᑳᑯᐧᐃᒡ, ᒥᒄ ᒫᒃ ᐧᐄᔭ ᑫᓂᕕᐢ ᑳᐦ ᓂᔥᑐᑎᐧᐃᔥᑖᔮᒡ ᑮᔮᐦ ᑳᐦ ᓈᐅᑎᐧᐃᔥᑖᔮᒡ ᐋᔥᒄ ᓈᔥᒡ ᒌᐦ ᒫᑯᐦᐄᑰ᙮ ᐊᓂᔮ ᑳ ᒥᔮᐅᐱᔭᔭᒡ ᐹᔭᑯᐲᓯᒻ, ᐋᑯᑎᐦ ᓈᔥᒡ ᑳ ᐧᐄᐦ ᒦᒋᑦ ᐊᓂᔮ ᒑᐧᑳᔮᐤ ᑳ ᒌ ᒦᒋᑦ, ᐋᑯᔥ ᒫᒃ ᑳᐦ ᒦᒋᑦ᙮ ᐊᐧᑳᑖᔮᐦᑎᐦᒃ ᐋᑯᔥ ᐋᑯᑖᐦ ᒑ ᐃᐦᑎᔮᓐ, ᓂᔮᓂᑯᑑᓐᐦ ᑳ ᒌ ᒦᒋᒡ ᐅᑎᐧᐋᔑᔒᒻᐦ ᐋᐦ ᐧᐄᒋᐦᐄᑯᑦ ᐋᑳ ᑭᔭᐧᐹ ᓈᔥᒡ ᐧᐄᐦ ᒫᑯᐦᐄᑯᑦ, ᒥᒄ ᒫᒃ ᒦᓐ ᑯᐃᔅᒄ ᑳ ᒌ ᐄᔑ ᒦᒋᓯᑦ᙮ ᑖᓐ ᒑ ᐃᐦᑎᔮᓐ ᐆ ᐃᐦᑐᑎᒫᓈ᙮ ᒥᒄ ᒫᒃ ᐊᓂᔮ ᑳ ᐄᔑ ᒫᑯᐦᐄᑯᑦ ᑳ ᐴᓂᐦᑖᑦ ᓂᑎᐧᐋ ᒑᐧᑳᔮᐤ ᐋᐦ ᒦᒋᑦ, ᒥᐦᒑᑐᐲᓯᒻ ᒌᐦ ᐱᒦᐦᑳᑯ᙮ ᑯᐧᑖᔥᒡ ᑎᐦᑐᐲᓯᒻ ᒌᐦ ᐱᒦᐦᑳᑯ᙮

ᐋᔪᐧᐃᒄ ᒫᒃ ᐅᔮ ᑳ ᒫᒥᑐᓈᔮᐦᑎᒥᐦᐄᑯᑦ ᒫᐧᑳᒡ ᐋᐦ ᐱᐹᒧᐦᑖᑦ᙮ ᐊᓂᒌ ᒫᒃ ᐧᐄ ᑯᑎᑭᒡ ᐊᐧᐋᓂᒌ ᒋᔅᒑᔮᐦᑎᒧᒐ ᒑᒃ ᐋᑳ ᒐ ᒌᐦ ᐴᓂᐦᑖᒡ ᔔᑳᔮᐤ ᐋᑦ ᐧᐄᐦ ᐴᓂᐦᑖᑖᐧᐋ᙮ ᓂᒥ ᐅᐦᒋ ᐹᐦᑎᐧᒫ ᑳ ᐋᔭᐧᒫᐅᐦᐄᐧᐋᔭᐧᑲ ᐊᓂᑖᐦ ᒋᔅᑯᑎᒫᑑᑭᒥᑯᐦᒡ᙮ ᐋᐧᐋ ᒥᒄ ᐧᐄᔭ ᐋᑖᔮᐦᑎᐦᒃ ᐋᐦ ᒦᒋᒥᐧᐃᔭᒡ

ᓯᔅᒋᑰᒡ ᐁ ᐴᓂᐦᑖᑦ ᒪᒋᓂᑐᐦᑯᐃᓂᔫ ᑲᔦ ᐁᑳ ᒥᔫᔅᑳᑫᔮᒡ ᒦᒋᒥᔪ ᐁᐅᒄ ᐅᔫ ᐧᐁᐦᒌ ᐃᔅᐸᔭᑦ ᐁ ᓇᓇᒥᐸᔭᑦ᙮ ᐁᑯᓐ ᐁ ᐃᔅᐸᔭᐧᑖᐤ ᒪᒋᓂᑐᐦᑯᐃᓂᔫ ᑲ ᐅᑎᓇᐦᐧᑳᐤ ᐦᐁᐧᓭᐧᐃᓐ ᑳ ᐃᓯᓂᐦᑳᑌᔭᒡ ᓯᔅᒋᑰᒡ ᒫᒃ ᐁ ᐴᓂᐦᑖᐧᑖᐤ᙮ ᐁᑎᑑ ᒫᒃ ᐃᔅᐸᔫᒡ, ᒥᐦᑫᑐ ᒌᔑᑳᐤ ᑕᔒᐦᑳᓯᒪᑲᓂᔫ ᑫᒌ ᐧᐄᐧᐄᐸᔭᔭᒡ ᐧᐄᔮᐦᒡ ᐊᐧᐁᓐ, ᐧᐃᔦᔅ ᐯᔭᒄ ᑑᔥᑌᐤ ᐃᔥᐱᔥ, ᐁᒄ ᐧᐄ ᑫᓂᕕᐢ ᓂᔥᑐ ᒫᒃ ᓄᐤ ᑑᔥᑌᐤ ᑳ ᐃᔥᐱᔥ ᐴᓂᐦᑖᑦ ᒦᒋᒥᔫ ᐁᑳ ᒥᔫᔅᑳᑫᒪᑲᓂᔭᒡ ᔮᐸᒡ ᓈᔅᒡ ᒌ ᓇᓇᒥᐸᔫ᙮ ᐯᔭᒄ ᐲᓯᒻ ᐁᑳ ᐅᐦᒋ ᒦᒋᑦ ᐊᓂᔫᐦ ᑫᐧᑳᔫᐦ ᑳᒌ ᒦᒋᑦ ᔮᐸᒡ ᒨᔥ ᒌᐧᐄ ᒦᒎ ᐁᒄ ᑮᐹ ᑳᒌ ᒦᒋᑦ᙮ ᐁᒄ ᑲ ᐃᑌᔭᐦᑕᒃ ᔮᐸᒡ ᑫᒌ ᑯᒋᐦᑖᑦ ᐁᑳ ᑫᒌ ᒦᒋᑦ ᐧᐁᔅ ᔖᔅ ᐯᔭᒄ ᐲᓯᒻ ᓂᒌ ᐅᑎᐦᑕᐦᐁᓐ ᒌ ᐃᑌᔭᐦᑕᒻ᙮ ᐯᔭᐧᑳᐤ ᒫᓐᐦ ᒉᔑᑯᒻ ᐲᓯᒻ ᐁ ᐅᑖᑯᔑᔭᒡ ᐅᑕᐧᐋᔒᒻ ᐁᒄ ᒫᒃ ᐧᐃᔭ ᒌ ᒦᒍᒡ ᐊᓂᔫᐦ ᑫᐧᑳᔫᐦ ᐁᑳ ᒥᔫᔅᑳᑫᒪᑲᓂᔭᐧᑳᐤᐦ᙮ ᐁᐅᒄ ᒥᒄ ᐊᓂᔫ ᐯᔭᐧᑳᐤ ᑳ ᐃᐦᑎᐧᑖᐤ ᐅᔫ, ᒌ ᒥᔦᔭᐦᑕᒻ ᒫᒃ ᐧᐁᔅ ᐅᔔ ᒨᔥ ᐁ ᒥᐧᔮᔑᔭᒡ ᒦᒋᒥᔫ ᒌ ᒨᒍᐤ ᒉᔑᑯᒻ ᐅᑖᑯᓰᐦ᙮ ᐃᐦᑕᑯᓐ ᐋ ᒫᒃ ᑫ ᐃᔑ ᒪᒋᑑᑖᑯᔮᓐ ᐆ ᐃᐦᑎᔮᓄ, ᒌ ᐃᑌᔭᐦᑕᒻ᙮ ᒋᓄᐅᔥ ᒌ ᑕᔒᐦᑳᓰ ᑫᓂᕕᐢ ᐁᐧᐄ ᐸᔦᐦᒋᐦᐄᓯᑦ, ᐅᔥᑌ ᐯᔭᒄ ᐲᓯᒻ, ᑫᒄ ᓃᔓ ᐲᓯᒻ ᒥᐦᑫᑐ ᐲᓯᒻ ᒌ ᑕᔒᐦᑳᑎᓰ᙮ ᐅᔥᑌ ᑯᐧᑖᔅᒡ ᐲᓯᒻ ᒌ ᐱᒥᐸᔭᓂᔫ ᔮᒄ ᑳ ᓇᑲᑎᑯᑦ ᐊᓂᔫ ᐁ ᐃᐦᑎᑦ ᒌ ᐋᔮᒥᐦᐄᑰ ᒫᒃ ᑖᐧᐯ᙮

ᐁᐅᒄ ᐅᔫ ᑳ ᒫᒥᑐᓄᔮᐦᑕᒥᐦᐄᑯᑦ ᐊᓂᔫ ᒫᓐᐦ ᐯᒧᐦᑌᒡ᙮ ᒋᔅᑫᔮᐦᑕᒧᒡ ᑳᑲᔦ ᐊᐧᐁᓂᒌ ᐅᑕ ᑳ ᐃᐦᑖᐧᑖᐤ ᐁ ᐃᔥᐱᔥ ᒫᔮᑕᓂᔮᒡ ᔔᑲᔫ, ᒥᒍᓐ ᑫᒌ ᑎᐯᔮᒥᑯᐧᑖᐤ ᑫᒌ ᐃᔑᓈᑯᓂᔮᒡ ᒌ ᐃᑌᔭᐦᑕᒻ᙮ ᒌ ᐋᔮᒨᑖᑲᓅᔫ ᐋ ᐊᓂᑌ ᒋᔅᑯᑕᒫᑫᐅᑲᒥᑯᐦᒡ ᐁᑳ ᒫᒃ ᐅᐦᒋ ᐯᐦᑕᒧᐧᑫ᙮

C'était un véritable sevrage. C'était ce que les héroïnomanes traversaient lorsqu'ils arrêtaient la poudre. Pire encore, puisque la désintoxication de l'héroïne durait quelques jours, une semaine tout au plus, alors qu'après trois semaines, puis quatre, les symptômes de désintoxication de Jennifer étaient toujours aussi forts. Après que le premier mois fut passé, elle avait toujours très envie de malbouffe, donc elle en mangea. Puis, elle se dit que puisqu'elle était arrivée jusque-là, autant continuer. Une fois par mois, elle passait donc une soirée malbouffe avec ses enfants pour ne pas se sentir privée, mais les autres soirs, elle pouvait tout aussi bien continuer à manger sainement. Qu'avait-elle à perdre ? Les symptômes de désintoxication de Jennifer, cependant, durèrent au-delà de ce premier mois et du mois suivant, et du mois suivant. Ils durèrent *six maudits mois*.

This was full-on addiction withdrawal. This was what heroin junkies went through when they went off smack. Worse, because heroin detox lasted a few days, a week at most and, after three weeks then four weeks, Jennifer's detox symptoms were still coming on strong. When the first month was up, she still really wanted junk food, so she had some. Then she figured she had come this far, might as well keep goin'. Once a month she would have a junk food night with her kids so that she wouldn't feel deprived, but the other nights she might as well keep on eating healthy. What did she have to lose? Jennifer's detox symptoms, though, lasted beyond that first month and the next and the next. They lasted for *six friggin' months*.

Elle y pensait en marchant. Les autres personnes des alentours savaient-elles que le sucre était une sacrée bonne vieille dépendance ? Avait-elle raté ce cours à l'école ? Était-elle la seule à avoir toujours pensé que la malbouffe était juste, vous

She thought about that as she walked. Did other folks around here know that sugar was a nasty ol' addiction? Had she missed that class in school? Was she the only one who had always thought junk food was, you know, *food*? Was she the only one

ᐊᓂᔮ ᓂᑎᐑ ᒑᒁᔨᐤ ᐋᐦ ᒦᒋᓈᓂᐎᐎᔨᒡ᙮
ᐋᐚ ᒥᒄ ᐑᔨ ᓂᒥ ᐅᐦᒋ ᒋᔅᒑᔨᐦᑎᒻ᙮

ᐹᔨᒁᐤ ᒫᒃ ᐋᐦ ᒑᒋᔖᐹᔭᔨᒡ, ᓈᓈᒑ ᐊᓂᔮ ᑳ ᐴᓂᐦᑖᑦ ᐋᐦ ᒦᒋᑦ ᓂᑎᐑ ᒑᒁᔨᐤ, ᓈᔥᒡ ᐋᑳ ᒥᔦᒥᒋᐦᐅᑦ ᐚᓂᔥᑳᑦ᙮ ᐋᐦ ᐋᐦᑯᔥᑎᒁᓈᑦ, ᐋᐦ ᐹᐦᐹᑯᒧᑦ, ᐋᐦ ᐹᔥᑖᔨᒡ ᐅᑐᓐ, ᒥᓯᐚ ᐋᑳ ᐄᔑ ᒥᒥᔦᒥᒋᐦᐅᑦ᙮

ᐋᑯᑖᐦ ᒥᒄ ᐋᔑ ᓂᐚᑳᐳᐎᓐ ᐊᓂᑖᐦ ᒦᓰᐅᑭᒥᑯᐦᒡ, ᐋᐦ ᐹᐦᐹᑭᒧᑦ, ᐋᐦ ᐹᐲᔨᐦᑖᑦ ᐊᓂᔮ ᒑᒁᔨᐤ ᐋᑳ ᒥᐧᔮᔨᒡ ᐊᓂᑖᐦ ᐅᑎᒋᔒᐦ ᑳᐦ ᐃᐦᑎᑯᓂᔨᒡ, ᑭᔮᐦ ᐋᐦ ᒫᒥᑐᓈᔨᐦᑎᐦᒃ᙮

ᒥᐦᒑᑖᐤ ᐋᐦ ᒌᐦ ᐄᑎᒥᒋᐦᐅᑦ ᐃᔅᑯᑎᒃ ᐴᓃᒡᐦ ᓈᐅᔥ ᐋᐦ ᒌᐦ ᒥᓂᐦᒁᑦ᙮ ᒎᔥ ᒫᒃ ᑳ ᐄᔥᐱᔑ ᒥᓂᐦᒁᑦ, ᓈᔥᒡ ᒑ ᒌᐦ ᒌᔥᒁᐹᑦ ᑭᔮᐦ ᐋᑳ ᒑ ᒋᔅᒋᓯᑦ, ᓃᔥᑎᓂᐚᐱᐳᓐᐦ ᐄᔥᐱᔥ, ᓃᔥᑎᒻ ᐊᓂᑖᐦ ᑳ ᐹᒋ ᓂᔮᓈᓈᐅᔖᐳᐳᐧᓈᓯᑦ᙮ ᓃᐧᔖᐤ ᑭᔮᐦ ᒫᒃ ᓂᔥᐧᑖᐤ ᐹᔨᑯᐲᓯᒻᐦ ᓃᔥᑎᓂᐚᐱᐳᓐᐦ ᐄᔥᐱᔥ =

ᓈᔥᑖᐧᐹᐦ ᒥᐦᒑᐧᑖᐤ ᒌᐦ ᐋᐦᑯᓵᐹᐧᐋᐤ᙮

ᒌᐦ ᔑᔥᑭᒋᐦᐄᑰ ᐋᐦ ᐋᐦᑯᓵᐹᐧᐋᑦ᙮ ᑭᔮᐦ ᐊᓂᔮ ᓈᔥᒡ ᐋᐦ ᒌᐦ ᒥᒑᔨᐦᑎᒦᔨᒡᐦ ᐅᑎᐧᐋᔑᔒᒻᐦ᙮

ᒥᒄ ᐋ ᐑᔭ ᒌ ᐃᐦᑖᐤ ᐁᒌ ᐃᑌᔨᐦᑕᒃ ᐁ ᒦᒋᒥᔅᑳᑫᔨᒡ ᒦᒋᒥᔫ ᐁᑳ ᑳ ᒦᒋᒉᔨᐦᑖᑯᓂᔨᒡ᙮ ᒥᒄ ᐋ ᐑᔭ ᒌ ᐯᔭᑯᔖ ᐁᑳ ᐅᐦᒋ ᒋᔅᒉᔨᐦᑕᐦᒃ ᐅᔫ᙮

ᐯᔭᒁᐤ ᐁ ᒉᒋᒐᐹᔭᔨᒡ, ᓵᔅ ᐌᔅᑳᒌᔒᔥ ᐁᒌ ᐴᓂᐦᑖᑦ ᐁᑳ ᒦᒋᒥᔅᑳᑫᔨᒡ ᒦᒋᒥᔫ ᐁ ᒦᒋᑦ, ᒌ ᐚᓂᔥᑳᐤ ᓈᔅᒡ ᐁ ᐋᐦᑯᔥᑎᒁᓄᑦ ᒨᐧᐁᐦᒡ ᐁᒌ ᒥᓂᐦᑵᑦ ᐁ ᐄᑕᒪᐦᒋᐦᐅᑦ᙮ ᒌ ᑌᐅᔥᑎᒁᓄᐤ, ᒌ ᐸᐹᐦᑯᒨ, ᒌ ᐹᐦᑯᑖᒨ, ᒥᓯᐌ ᑳᒌ ᐃᑕᒪᐦᒋᐅᑦ ᐊᐧᐁᓐ ᐁᒌ ᒥᓂᐦᑵᑦ ᐁᑯᓐ ᑳ ᐃᑕᒪᐦᒋᐦᐅᑦ᙮

ᒦᓰᐅᔮᑲᓂᐦᒡ ᐁ ᐃᔑ ᓇᐧᐁᐱᑦ ᐁ ᐹᐦᐹᑯᒧᑦ ᒌ ᒫᒥᑐᓄᔨᐦᑕᒻ ᑖᓐ ᐁ ᐃᔅᐸᔨᑦ᙮

ᑖᐧᐯᐦ ᒥᐦᒉᐧᑖᐤ ᒫᓐᐦ ᒌ ᐋᐦᑯᓯᐧᐋᐹᐧᐁᐤ᙮ ᓃᔥᑐᓅ ᐱᐳᓐ ᐁᑯᓐ ᑳ ᐃᔑᓈᑯᓯᑦ ᐱᔑᒄ ᐁᒌ ᒥᓂᐦᑵᑦ, 18 ᒌ ᑕᐦᑐᐳᓄᓰ ᑳ ᒋᐦᒋᐸᔨᐦᑖᑦ ᐅᔫ ᐁ ᐄᑖᑎᓰᑦ᙮ ᓃᐧᔖᐤ ᐋᔅᑰ ᓂᔥᐧᑖᐤ ᐯᔭᒄ ᐲᓯᒻᐦ ᐁᒌ ᒥᓂᐦᑵᑦ ᑲᔦ ᐋᔅᑰ ᐁᑎᑑ ᒥᐦᒉᐧᑖᐤ ᒌ ᒥᓂᐦᑵᐤ᙮

ᓈᓂᑑ ᐅᔥᑌ ᐯᔭᒁᐤ ᒋᒐᒥᑖᐦᑐᓂᑐᓄᐧᐋᐤ ᒌ ᐋᐦᑯᓯᐧᐋᐹᐧᐁᒉ᙮

ᐁᒄ ᒫᒃ ᒉᒃ ᑳ ᓯᔅᑲᒋᐦᐄᑯᑦ ᐅᔫ ᐁ ᐃᐦᑎᑦ᙮ ᓄᔅᑕ ᑲᔦ ᐅᑕᐧᐋᔑᔒᒻᐦ ᒌ ᓯᔅᑲᒋᐦᐁᐤ ᐁ

savez, de la *bouffe* ? Était-elle la seule à ne pas l'avoir su ?

who had never known?

Un matin, un moment après avoir cessé de manger de la malbouffe, Jennifer se réveilla avec une sacrée gueule de bois. Maux de tête, vomissements, bouche sèche, la totale.

One morning, a while after she had quit junk food, Jennifer woke with a bad-ass hangover. Headache, puking, dry mouth, the works.

Elle était ainsi penchée au-dessus de la cuvette, aux prises des haut-le-cœur de ses tripes malheureuses, et elle réfléchissait.

She hung over the toilet, heaving out the dregs of her unhappy gut, and thinking.

Elle avait sans aucun doute eu beaucoup de gueules de bois de son temps.
Elle avait bu avec la même intensité, l'intensité de l'adolescente qui essaie de s'en mettre une bonne, pendant vingt ans, depuis qu'elle avait 18 ans. Deux ou trois fois par mois pendant vingt ans, avec quelques années de consommation particulièrement intense en cours de route –

She sure had had plenty of hangovers in her day. She had been drinking at the same level, the teenager-trying-to-get-good and-wasted level, for twenty years, since she had been 18 years old. Two or three times a month for twenty years plus a few extra-intense years along the way –

Plus de *mille* gueules de bois.

Over a *thousand* hangovers.

Elle en avait marre des gueules de bois. Et de la façon dont son alcoolisme

She was sick of hangovers. And of how her drinking upset her kids. When she

ᐊᓂᑖᐦ ᐧᐋᔨᐧᐄᒡᐦ ᒑ ᓂᑑᒥᓂᐦᐧᑳᑦ, ᐊᓂᔫᐦ ᒑᔖᔨᔨᐅᐧᐃᔑᔨᒡᐦ ᐋᓯᐧᐃᑯᓐᐦ ᑳ ᒌ ᓂᑭᑎᒧᐧᐋᑦ ᐊᓂᔫᐦ ᐋᐧᐋᔑᔒᐧᐃᔑᔨᒡᐦ ᒑ ᑭᓂᐧᐋᔨᒫᔨᒡᐦ, ᑭᔫᐦ ᓈᔥᒡ ᐋᐦ ᒌᐦ ᒥᒑᔨᐦᑎᒥᔨᒡᐦ ᐊᓂᔫᐦ ᒑᔖᔨᔨᐧᐃᔑᔨᒡᐦ ᐋᑳ ᐅᐦᒋ ᐃᔫᐱᓯᐦᑖᑯᔨᒡᐦ ᐊᓂᔫᐦ ᐅᔒᒥᔑᔨᐤᐦ᙮ ᒥᓯᐧᐋ ᐊᐧᐋᓐ ᒌᐦ ᐋᔨᒥᔨᑰ, ᒥᓯᐧᐋ ᐊᐧᐋᓐ᙮

ᐋᑰ ᒫᒃ, ᐄᑖᔨᐦᑎᒻ ᒉᓂᕕᕐ, ᐊᓂᑖᐦ ᒦᓰᐅᑭᒥᑯᐦᒡ ᐋᐦ ᐄᑎᔅᐧᑳᔨᑦ᙮ ᐋᑰ ᒫᒃ᙮

ᔖᔥ ᒋᔅᒑᔨᐦᑎᒻ ᐊᓂᑖᐦ ᒑ ᐃᐦᑎᒃ᙮ ᒋᑭ ᑯᒋᔥᑖᐤ ᐹᔨᑯᐲᓯᒻᐦ ᐋᑳ ᒐ ᐱᒫᔨᐦᑎᐦᒃ ᑳᒥᓂᐦᐧᑳᓂᐧᐃᐧᐃᔨᒡ᙮ ᐆᐧᐊ, ᓂᒧᐃ ᑭᔨᐧᐹ ᐋᑳ ᓈᔥᑎᔨᒻ ᐱᒫᔨᐦᑎᐦᒃ = ᑖᐹ ᓂᒥᔫᔨᐤ ᐅᑎᐦ ᐋᐦ ᐧᐄᐦ ᔫᓃᑦ ᐊᐧᐋᓐ ᐋᐦ ᒥᓂᐦᐧᑳᑦ ᐋᐦ ᐄᑐᐦᑖᑦ ᒫᓐᐦ ᐋᐦ ᓂᔥᑎᐧᐄᓈᓂᐧᐃᐧᐃᔨᒡ᙮ ᐧᑳᐧᔖᓐ ᒥᒄ ᐹᔨᑯᒥᓂᐦᐧᑳᑭᓐ ᐹᔨᐧᑳᐤ ᐋᐦ ᑎᐧᐃᔥᑖᔨᒡ, ᐹᐦᑳᒡ ᒥᒄ ᐋᐦ ᒥᓂᐦᐧᑳᑦ, ᐹᔨᒄ ᐲᓯᒻ ᐋᑳ ᓈᔥᒡ ᒥᔥᒌᐦ ᒐ ᒥᓂᐦᐧᑳᑦ, ᑭᔫᐦ ᓂᒧᐃ ᐋᔑᑯᒥᑎᐧᐃᔥᑖᐤᐦ ᒐ ᒌᐦ ᒥᓂᐦᐧᑳᑦ ᑯᐧᑖᔥᒡ ᑳ ᐲᔥᒑᐅᐱᔑᔨᒡᐦ ᐋᔑᑯᒥᑎᐱᔅᑳᐤᐦ᙮

ᑭᔫᐦ ᒫᒃ, ᓂᒧᐃ ᔖᔥ ᓈᔥᒡ ᓂᑎᐧᐋᔨᐦᑎᒻ᙮ ᐊᓅᐦᒡ ᒫᒃ ᓂᒧᐃ ᐹᐦᑎᐧᐋᐤ ᐊᓂᔫᐦ ᑳ ᐅᐧᐹᔨᒥ ᐋᐦ ᒫᐦᒫᔨᐦᒋᑎᑯᑦ, ᐋᑳ ᑭᔨᐧᐹ ᔖᔥ ᒨᔥ ᒥᒋᒥᒋᐦᐅᑦ, ᓂᒧᐃ ᓂᑎᐧᐋᔨᐦᑎᒻ ᒑᐧᑳᔨᐤ ᒐ ᒌᐦ ᐧᐄᒋᐦᐄᑯᑦ ᐋᑳ ᒐ ᒌᐦ ᐹᐦᑎᐧᐋᑦ᙮ ᓈᓈᓂᒌᒻ ᒫᒃ ᐊᑎ ᒥᐧᔫᔨᐦᑎᒻ ᐅᐱᒫᑎᓰᐧᐃᓐ, ᐃᐦᑎᑯᓂᔨᐤ ᒐᐧᑳᔨᐤ ᒐ ᐅᐦᒋ ᐱᒫᑎᓯᑦ᙮

ᒥᓂᐦᐧᑫᑦ᙮ ᒣᓂᐦᐧᑫᒡ ᒌ ᓇᑲᑌᐤ ᐊᓂᓰᐦ ᑳ ᐋᔫᐱᔒᔑᐧᑖᐤ ᐅᑕᐧᐋᔒᒻ ᒉᒌ ᑲᓇᐧᐁᔨᒥᑯᔨᒡ ᐊᓂᓰᐦ ᓃᔥᑕᒻ ᑳ ᐋᔫᐧᐋᑦ ᐊᐧᐋᔕ᙮ ᓵᔅ ᑮᐹ ᒌ ᐃᔅᐱᐦᑖᑎᓯᓰᐦ ᒉᒌ ᑲᓇᐧᐋᒉᔨᒡ ᒥᒄ ᒫᒃ ᓇᒧᐃ ᐅᐦᒋ ᒥᔐᔨᐦᑕᒧᒡ ᐊᓂᒌ ᑯᑕᑲᒡ ᐊᐧᐋᔕᒡ ᐧᐁᓵ ᐁ ᐧᐄ ᐃᐦᑑᑖᑯᐧᑖᐤ ᐊᓂᓰᐦ ᑳ ᑲᓇᐧᐁᔨᒥᑯᐧᑖᐤ ᐁᒄ ᐊᓐ ᑳ ᑲᓇᐧᐁᔨᒫᑦ ᐅᔒᒻᐦ ᓇᒧᐃ ᐅᐦᒋ ᒥᔐᔨᐦᑕᒻ ᐁᑳ ᐱᓯᒋᐦᐄᑯᑦ᙮ ᒥᓯᐧᐁ ᒌ ᐋᔨᒥᐦᐄᑰᒡ ᑖᓐ ᐁ ᐃᔅᐸᔨᐧᑖᐤ ᐊᓂᑕᐦ ᐧᐄᒋᐧᐋᐧᐋᐦᒡ᙮

ᐊᓂᓰ ᒫᒃ ᒣᐧᑳᒡ ᐊᓂᑌ ᒦᓰᐅᑲᒥᑯᐦᒡ ᐁ ᐊᐱᑦ, ᐁᑯᓐ ᐁᒄ, ᒌ ᐅᐦᒋ ᐃᑌᔨᐦᑕᒻ ᒉᓂᕕᕐ᙮

ᐁᑯᑦ ᑳ ᐅᐦᒋ ᒋᔅᒉᔨᐦᑕᐦᒃ ᒉ ᐃᐦᑎᑦ᙮ ᒋᑲ ᑯᒋᐦᑖᐤ ᐯᔨᒄ ᐲᓯᒻ ᐁᑳ ᒥᓂᐦᐧᑫᑦ᙮ ᓇᒧᐃ ᑮᐹ ᓈᓂᑑ ᐁᑳ ᒥᒍᓐ ᒥᓂᐦᐧᑫᑦ ᐧᐁᔅ ᑖᐹ ᐃᐦᑕᑯᓐ ᑖᓂᑌ ᒉ ᐅᐦᒋ ᓇᓈᑲᒋᐦᐄᑯᔫᓐ ᒌ ᐃᑌᔨᐦᑕᒻ᙮ ᐋᔥᑰ ᓂᑲ ᒥᓂᐦᐧᑫᔑᓐ ᒥᒄ ᐊᐱᔒᔥ ᒣᔑᑯᒻ ᑑᔥᑌᐤᐦ, ᒌ ᐃᑌᔨᐦᑕᒻ ᒥᒄ ᓇᒧᐃ ᓂᑲ ᐅᐦᒋ ᒌᔥᐧᑫᐯᓐ᙮ ᓇᒧᐃ ᐧᐄ ᑯᐧᑖᔅᒡ ᔫᑕᐃ ᓂᑲ ᐅᐦᒋ ᒥᓂᐦᐧᑫᓐ ᑳᒌ ᐃᐦᑎᔫᓐ ᒣᔑᑯᒻ ᐅᑖᑯᔖᐦ ᒌ ᐃᑌᔨᐦᑕᒻ᙮

ᓇᒧᐃ ᑮᐹ ᓵᔅ ᐅᐦᒋ ᐃᔥᐱᔥ ᓂᑐᐧᐁᔨᐦᑕᒻ᙮ ᓇᒧᐃ ᐅᐦᒋ ᐃᐦᑖᓰ ᐅᐧᐄᐦᐧᑫᔫᒻ ᒉᒌ ᒫᔐᔨᒥᑯᑦ ᑲᔐ ᓇᒧᐃ ᐅᐦᒋ ᐋᐦᑯᓯᓰ ᒨᔥ ᐁᒄ ᒫᒃ ᓇᒧᐃ ᐅᐦᒋ ᓂᑐᐧᐁᔨᐦᑕᒻ ᒉᐧᑳᓰ᙮ ᐧᐁᑖᒡ ᒌ ᒨᔑᐦᑖᐤ ᐋᐦᒌᐅᐦ ᐁ ᐃᑌᔨᒧᑦ, ᒌᐧᐄ ᐱᒫᑎᓰᐤ᙮

contrariait ses enfants. Quand elle sortait boire, elle laissait les cadets à la garde de l'aîné, qui était assez âgé pour les surveiller, mais les cadets n'appréciaient pas que l'aîné soit en charge, et l'aîné détestait être mis dans la position difficile de surveiller des enfants plus jeunes qui refusaient de l'écouter. C'était une situation difficile pour tous et chacun, à tous les niveaux.

*C'est fini*, pensa Jennifer en regardant dans la cuvette des toilettes. *Plus jamais.*

Désormais, elle savait quoi faire. Elle pouvait passer un mois sans alcool. Peut-être pas totalement sans, en fait - on n'était pas dans les AA. Elle savourerait un verre de quelque chose toutes les semaines environ, le siroterait lentement; mais pendant un mois, elle ne se soûlerait plus et elle ne boirait plus de pack de six bières chaque soir.

De plus, elle n'en avait plus autant besoin. Puisqu'elle n'avait plus à écouter son ex l'insulter, puisque son corps ne se sentait plus tout le temps malade désormais, elle n'avait plus besoin de s'échapper. Sa vie commençait à ressembler à quelque chose qui valait la peine d'être vécu, une

went out drinking, she would leave the younger kids in the care of the eldest, who was old enough to babysit, but the younger ones resented having the oldest be the boss of them, and the oldest hated being in that difficult position with younger kids who wouldn't listen. It was hard for everybody, all around.

*That's it,* Jennifer thought, looking into the toilet bowl. *No more.*

Now she knew what to do. She could do one month without booze. Well, maybe not totally without – this wasn't AA. She would savor a glass of something every week or so, sip it slowly, but for a month there would be no more getting wasted, and no more six-pack of beer every evening.

Besides, she didn't need it so much. Now that she didn't have to listen to her ex hurling insults at her, now that her body didn't feel sick all the time, she didn't need escape. Her life was beginning to feel like something worth living, something worth sticking around for.

ᐊᓂᔮ ᒫᒃ ᒑᑳᑦ ᓈᔥᑎᔨᒡ ᐋᑳ ᒥᓂᐦᐧᑳᑦ ᓂᒧᐃ ᐅᐦᒋ ᐧᐋᐦᑎᓂᔨᐤ = ᓈᔥᒡ ᐋᐦ ᒌᐦ ᒫᑯᐦᐄᑯᑦ ᒫᓐ ᐋᐦ ᐧᐄᐦ ᒥᓂᐦᐧᑳᑦ ᑮᔮᐦ ᐹᔨᑯᐲᓯᒻᐦ ᐊᓂᔮ ᒌᐦ ᐃᐦᑎᐤ, ᑮᔮᐦ ᒦᓐ ᓂᔮᓂᑯᑑᓐᐦ ᒫᓐ ᑳ ᒌ ᐧᐄᐦ ᒥᓂᐦᐧᑳᑦ = ᒥᒄ ᒫᒃ ᓂᒧᐃ ᐅᐦᒋ ᔖᑯᐦᐄᑰ᙮ ᐊᓂᔮ ᒫᒃ ᑳ ᐋᑎ ᐄᔥᐧᑳᑯᒥᓃᔨᒡᐦ ᐲᓯᒻᐦ ᓈᔥᑎᔨᒡ ᓂᒥ ᐅᐦᒋ ᐋᐦᑯᓵᐹᐧᐋᐤ, ᒌᐦ ᒥᐧᔮᔨᐦᑎᒻ ᒫᒃ ᐅᔮ ᐋᑳ ᐋᐦᑯᓯᑦ ᑮᔮᐦ ᓂᒥ ᒦᓐ ᐅᐦᒋ ᐧᐄᐦ ᒥᓂᐦᐧᑳᐤ᙮

ᓂᒧᐃ ᑭᔨᐧᐹ ᓈᔥᑎᔨᒡ ᐅᐦᒋ ᐴᓃᐤ = ᓂᒧᐃ ᐅᐦᒋ ᒥᔫᐦᑎᒻ ᐊᓂᔮ ᐴᓃᐤ ᐋᐦ ᐄᓈᓂᐧᐃᐧᐃᔨᒡ ᒧᔮᒻ ᐊᓂᑖᐦ ᐋᐦ ᐄᑎᐦᑎᐦᒃ ᒦᓐ ᒑ ᒋᔥᒌᑦ ᐋᐦ ᒥᓂᐦᐧᑳᑦ, ᐧᒫᐦᒡ ᐊᓂᔮ ᐋᐦ ᐄᐦᑎᔨᒡᐦ ᐊᐧᐋᔨᐤᐦ ᒥᒄ ᐧᐋᔨᐱᔥᒌᔥ ᐋᐦ ᐴᓃᒡᐦ ᐋᐦ ᐲᐦᐧᑖᔨᒡᐦ ᒦᓐ ᒫᒃ ᐹᑎᒫᐦ ᐋᐦ ᐱᐦᐧᑖᔨᒡᐦ᙮ ᒥᒄ ᒫᒃ ᐧᐄᔨ ᒋᔥᒋᐧᐋ ᒌᐦ ᐴᓃᐤ᙮ ᓈᔥᑎᔨᒡ ᒌᐦ ᐴᓃᐤ᙮ ᓈᔥᑎᔨᒡ ᒌᐦ ᐴᓂᐦᑖᐤ᙮ ᓂᒧᐃ ᒦᓐ ᒋᑭ ᐅᐧᐃᑎᓂᒻ᙮

ᓂᒧᐃ ᒦᓐ ᒥᐦᒑᑐᒌᔑᑳᐤᐦ ᒋᑭ ᒥᓂᐦᐧᑳᐤ ᑮᔮᐦ ᓂᒧᐃ ᒦᓐ ᒋᑭ ᐋᐦᑯᓵᐹᐧᐋᐤ ᒑ ᐄᔥᐱᔑ ᐱᒫᑎᓰᑦ᙮

ᓂᒧᐃ ᓈᔥᒡ ᓈᐅᔥ ᑳ ᐴᓃᑦ ᐋᐦ ᒥᓂᐦᐧᑳᑦ, ᒉᓂᕕᕝ ᒌᐦ ᐄᑐᐦᑖᐤ ᐊᓂᑖᐦ ᓂᑐᐦᑯᔨᓂᑭᒥᑯᐦᒡ ᒑ ᓂᑑᑎᐹᔨᒫᑭᓂᐧᐃᑦ ᐅᐦᒋ ᐊᓂᔮ ᐋᐦ ᔖᑳᐅᐱᔨᑦ᙮ ᐋᔮᐱᒡ ᐊᐧᑳᐦᑎᔨᒡᐦ ᐊᓂᔮᐦ ᑳ ᐧᐄᒋᐦᐋᔨᒡᐦ ᐊᐧᐋᔨᐤᐦ ᐊᑎᑎᐤ ᒑ ᒌᐦ ᒥᔫᒦᒋᓯᔨᒡᐦ ᓈᔥᒡ ᓈᐅᔥ ᐋᐦ ᐋᔨᒦᔨᒡᐦ᙮ ᒌᐦ

ᓇᒧᐃ ᑮᐹ ᐅᐦᒋ ᐧᐁᐦᑕᓂᔫ ᒋᐦᒋᐧᐁ ᒉᒌ ᐴᓃᑦ ᐁ ᒥᓂᐦᐧᑫᑦ = ᒥᒍᓐ ᐯᔨᒄ ᐲᓯᒻ ᐱᔑᒄ ᒌ ᐃᑌᔨᐦᑕᒻ ᒉᒌ ᒥᓂᐦᐧᑫᑦ ᑳ ᒪᔅᑲᐧᐋᑲᒥᔨᒡ ᐁᒄ ᒉᒃ ᒥᒄ ᐋᔥᑰ ᒌ ᒨᔑᐦᑖᐤ ᐁᐧᐄ ᒥᓂᐦᐧᑫᑦ = ᐁᑯᓐ ᑳ ᐃᔅᐸᔨᑦ᙮ ᐃᔅᑯᑕᒃ ᐯᔨᒄ ᐲᓯᒻ ᒉᔫᐅᐸᔨᓂᔨᒡ ᐁᑳ ᐅᐦᒋ ᐋᐦᑯᓯᐧᐋᐹᐧᐁᑦ, ᒌ ᒥᔦᔨᐦᑕᒻ ᐅᔫ ᐁᒄ ᓇᒧᐃ ᒦᓐ ᓂᐦᑖ ᐅᐦᒋ ᐧᐄ ᒥᔅᑕᒥᓂᐦᐧᑫᐤ ᒉᒌ ᐋᐦᑯᓯᐧᐋᐹᐧᐁᑦ᙮

ᓇᒧᐃ ᐅᐦᒋ ᐃᑌᔨᐦᑕᒻ ᓂᑲ ᐴᓃᓐ ᐁ ᒥᓂᐦᐧᑫᔮᓐ = ᓇᒧᐃ ᐅᐦᒋ ᒥᔫᐦᑕᒻ ᐅᔫ ᐁ ᐃᐧᑌᑦ ᐊᐧᐁᓐ ᐧᐁᔥ ᒧᐧᐁᐦᒡ ᒦᓐ ᒉ ᒋᐦᒋᐸᔨᐦᑖᑦ ᐁ ᒥᓂᐦᐧᑫᑦ ᒌ ᐄᑎᐦᑕᒻ, ᒧᐧᐁᐦᒡ ᐊᐧᐁᓐ ᓃᔓᑑᔥᑌᐤᐦ ᑳ ᐴᓃᑦ ᐁ ᐲᐦᐧᑖᑦ ᒦᓐ ᒫᒃ ᐁ ᐲᐦᐧᑖᑦ᙮ ᓂᑲ ᐴᓂᐦᑖᐦ ᒌ ᐃᑌᐤ ᐧᐄᔨ᙮ ᑌᑲᔥ ᓂᑲ ᐴᓂᐦᑖᓐ᙮ ᐁᑯᓐ ᐁᒄ᙮

ᓇᒧᐃ ᒦᓐ ᒥᐦᒉᑐ ᒌᔑᑳᐤ ᓂᑲ ᐅᐦᒋ ᒥᓂᐦᐧᑫᓐ ᑲᔦ ᓇᒧᐃ ᒦᓐ ᓂᑲ ᐅᐦᒋ ᐋᐦᑯᓯᐧᐋᐹᐧᐁᓐ ᒉ ᐃᔥᐱᔥ ᐱᒫᑎᓰᐧᐋᓐ, ᒌ ᐃᑌᔨᐦᑕᒻ᙮

ᐃᔅᑯᑕᒃ ᒫᒃ ᑳ ᐴᓂᐦᑖᑦ ᐃᔅᑯᑌᐧᐋᔨᔫ, ᓂᑐᐦᑯᐃᓂᑲᒥᑯᐦᒡ ᒌ ᐃᑐᐦᑌᐤ ᒉᒌ ᓂᑑ ᒋᔅᒉᔨᒫᑲᓅᑦ ᐊᓂᔫ ᐁ ᔫᐧᐋᑲᒥᐦᐧᑫᑦ᙮ ᐁᒄ ᑮᐹ ᒦᓐ ᑳ ᐊᔨᒥᐦᐄᑯᑦ ᐊᓂᔫᐦ ᑳ ᐧᐧᐋᐧᐄᐦᑕᒫᑯᑦ ᒉ ᐃᔑ ᓇᓈᑲᒋᐦᑖᑦ ᐁ ᐃᔑ ᒦᒋᓯᑦ᙮ ᐸᔅᒡ ᐊᓂᔫ ᑳ ᐃᐧᑌᔨᒡ ᓇᒧᐃ ᐅᐦᒋ ᓂᓯᑐᐦᑕᐧᐁᐤ ᑖᓐ ᐁ

chose pour laquelle ça valait la peine de rester dans les parages.

Cesser presque complètement de boire ne fut pas tout à fait facile – elle eut de fortes envies d'alcool pendant un mois et de légères envies pendant quelques mois par la suite – toutefois, c'était gérable. Et, vous savez quoi ? Au bout d'un mois sans une seule gueule de bois, elle aimait la façon dont elle se sentait et ne voulait plus se saouler à nouveau.

Cutting out most drinking wasn't exactly easy – she had heavy liquor cravings for a month, and light cravings for a few months after that – but it was manageable. And wouldn't you know, at the end of a month without a single hangover, she liked how she felt and didn't want to get wasted again.

Elle *n'arrêtait* pas – elle n'aimait pas ce mot parce qu'*arrêter* donnait l'impression qu'elle allait peut-être recommencer, comme les gens qui arrêtaient de fumer pendant quelques semaines et qui recommençait. Elle *cessait*. Point final. Fini. Plus jamais.

She wasn't *quitting* – she didn't like that word because *quitting* sounded like she might begin again, like the folks who quit smoking for a couple of weeks and then took it up again. She was *stopping*. Full *stop*. Done. No more.

Plus aucune cuite ou gueule de bois de toute sa vie.

Not another binge or hangover in her entire life.

Peu après avoir cessé de boire de l'alcool, Jennifer se rendit à la clinique pour son suivi du diabète. La nutritionniste parla encore et encore. Elle utilisait des termes scientifiques et puis Jennifer était censée faire ceci et pas cela; et elle faisait ci et

Soon after the end of booze, Jennifer went to the clinic for her diabetes follow-up. The nutritionist went on and on again. There were some Science words and then Jennifer was supposed to do this and not supposed to do that and she was

ᐋᐱᒥᔥᑖᔭᐤᐦ ᐊᔭᒧᐧᐃᓐᐦ ᐋᑳ ᐅᐦᒋ ᓂᓯᑐᐦᑎᐦᒃ ᑭᔮᐦ ᑳ ᐄᑎᑯᑦ ᒫᐤ ᔮᔭᑖ ᒑ ᐃᐦᑐᑎᒥᓐ ᑭᔮᐦ ᒫᐤ ᔮᔭᑖ ᓂᒥ ᒋᑭ ᐃᐦᑐᑖ ᑭᔮᐦ ᐋᐦ ᐄᑎᑯᑦ ᒫᐤ ᓂᒥ ᑯᐃᔅᒄ ᐊᔥᑎᐦᑎᓐ ᑭᔮᐦ ᒫᒃ ᐋᐅᒄ ᐆ ᒦᓐ ᓂᒥ ᑯᐃᔅᒄ ᐊᔥᑎᐦᑎᓐ ᑭᔮᐦ ᐊᑎᑎᐤ ᒑ ᒦᒌᓐ ᐆ ᑭᔮᐦ ᐋᑲᐧᐄ ᒥᔥᒌᐦ ᒦᒡᐦ ᐆ ᑭᔮᐦ ᒥᒄ ᐋᔥᐱᔑᔭᒡᐦ ᓈᔥᒡ ᒥᔥᒌᐦ ᐋᐦ ᐋᔭᒥᐦᐄᑯᑦ᙮

ᑳᐦ ᒌᐧᐋᑦ ᐊᓂᑖᐦ ᐅᐦᒋ ᓂᑐᐦᑯᔭᓂᑭᒥᑯᐦᒡ ᑭᔮᐦ ᑳᐦ ᒫᒥᑐᓈᔭᐦᑎᐦᒃ ᐊᓂᔮ ᑲ ᐄᑖᑭᓂᐧᐃᑦ᙮

ᑖᐧᐹᐦ ᐋ, ᐱᔑᔑᒄ ᐊᓂᔮ ᐋᑳ ᒥᔪᐦᑖᑯᓂᔭᒡ ᐋᔪᐧᐃᒄ ᑳᐦ ᐄᑖᑭᓂᐧᐃᑦ ᑭᔮᐦ ᒥᒄ ᒌᐦ ᐅᐧᐋᓈᔭᐦᑎᒥᐦᐄᑰ ᑭᔮᐦ ᓈᔥᑎᔭᒡ ᓂᒥ ᐅᐦᒋ ᐧᐄᒋᐦᐄᑰ᙮ ᑖᐹ ᐅᐦᒋ ᓂᑎᐧᐋᔭᒫᐤ ᒥᒄ ᐊᓂᔮ ᐋᑳ ᑯᐃᔅᒄ ᐃᔭᐦᑎᒃ ᒑ ᐧᐄᐦ ᑎᒫᑯᑦ ᐊᐧᐋᔭᐤᐦ ᑭᔮᐦ ᒑᐧᑳᔭᐤ ᒑ ᒦᒋᑦ ᑭᔮᐦ ᒫᒃ ᐧᐋᔅ ᐋᐦ ᑖᐦᒋᐳᑦ = ᐋᔪᐧᐃᒄ ᒨᔥ ᑳ ᒌ ᐹᐦᑎᐧᐋᑦ ᐊᓂᔮᐦ ᑳ ᐱᐱᒋᔅᑭᓈᐱᔭᒡᐦ ᐋᐦ ᐄᑎᑯᑦ ᑭᔮᐦ ᔖᔥ ᓂᒥ ᐧᐄᐦ ᐹᐦᑎᒻ ᐊᓂᔮ᙮

ᐋᑰ ᒫᒃ, ᐄᑖᔭᐦᑎᒻ, ᓂᒧᐃ ᒦᓐ ᓂᑭᓂᑎᐧᐋᐱᒫᐤ ᐊᓐ ᓂᑐᐦᑯᔭᓂᔅᐧᑳᐤ ᑲ ᐧᐋᐧᐄᐦᑎᒧᐧᐋᑦ ᐊᐧᐋᔭᐤᐦ ᒑ ᐄᔑ ᒦᒋᓱᔭᒡᐦ, ᓂᒧᐃ ᒦᓐ ᓂᑭ ᐃᔭᑐᐦᑖᓐ ᐊᓂᑖᐦ ᐋᐦ ᐅᐦᒋ ᓈᓈᑭᒥᐦᐋᑭᓂᐅᐧᐃᒡ ᐊᐧᐋᓂᒌ ᐋᐦ ᔖᑳᐅᐱᔭᒡ᙮ ᐊᔮᐱᒡ ᑭᑎ ᐃᐦᑐᑎᒻ ᐊᓂᔮ ᒑᐧᑳᔭᐤ ᐋ ᐃᐦᑐᑎᐦᒃ ᐋᐦ ᒥᔪᒥᒋᐦᐅᑦ ᑭᔮᐦ ᓂᒧᐃ ᑭᑎ ᐃᐦᑐᑎᒻ ᐊᓂᔮ ᒑᐧᑳᔭᐤ ᓈᔥᒡ ᐋᐦ ᒥᒑᔭᐦᑎᒥᐦᐄᑯᑦ᙮ ᑭᔭᐧᐹ ᒑ ᓂᑎᐧᐋᐱᒫᑦ ᐋᔅᑰ ᓂᑐᐦᑯᔭᓐᐦ, ᐊᓂᔮ ᑭᔭᐧᐹ ᒨᔥ ᑳ ᒌ ᐃᐦᑎᒃ᙮ ᒥᒄ ᓂᒧᐃ ᑭᑎ ᐃᔭᑐᐦᑖᐤ ᐊᓂᑖᐦ ᐋᐦ ᓂᑑᑎᐹᔭᒫᑭᓂᐧᐃᐧᐃᔭᒡᐦ ᐊᐧᐋᔭᐤᐦ ᐋᐦ ᔖᑳᐅᐱᔭᔭᒡᐦ᙮

ᐃᑎᑯᑦ ᑲᔦ ᒫᐤ ᒉ ᐃᐦᑎᔭᓐ, ᑲᔦ ᒫᐤ ᐁᑳ ᒉ ᐅᐦᒋ ᐃᐦᑎᔭᓐ ᑲᔦ ᒌ ᐧᐄᐦᑕᒫᑰ ᑖᓐ ᐁ ᐃᔑ ᐁᑳ ᒧᔮᒻ ᐃᐦᑎᑦ ᑲᔦ ᒌ ᐧᐄᐦᑕᒫᑰ ᒉᐧᑳᔫ ᒋᐹ ᒦᒎ, ᓈᔅᒡ ᒥᔅᑕᐦᐄ ᐁᒌᔑ ᐧᐋᐧᐄᐦᑕᒫᑯᑦ ᐁᑳ ᑖᐧᐯ ᐧᐄ ᓂᑐᐦᑕᐧᐋᑦ᙮

ᐊᓂᔫ ᒫᒃ ᐁ ᐊᑎ ᒌᐧᐁᑦ ᒌ ᒫᒥᑐᓀᔭᐦᑕᒻ ᐅᔫ᙮

ᑖᐧᐯ ᑮᐹ, ᒌ ᓃᐦᑕᐦᐆᑰ ᑖᓐ ᑳ ᐃᔑ ᐯᐦᑕᐦᒃ ᑲᔦ ᒌ ᐧᐊᐧᐋᓀᔭᐦᑕᒥᐦᐄᑰ, ᓇᒧᐃ ᐅᐦᒋ ᐧᐄᒋᐦᐄᑰ᙮ ᓇᒧᐃ ᐅᐦᒋ ᐧᐄ ᐯᐦᑕᐧᐁᐤ ᐊᐧᐁᔫ ᐁ ᐧᐋᐧᐄᐦᑕᒫᑯᑦ ᑖᓂᑕᐦ ᐁ ᐧᐊᓂᐸᔭᑦ ᑲᔦ ᒉ ᐃᔑ ᒦᒋᓱᑦ ᑲᔦ ᒋᑖᐦᒋᐳᓐ ᒉᒌ ᐄᑎᑯᑦ = ᐧᐁᔅ ᐁᑯᓐ ᑳᒌ ᐃᔑ ᐊᔭᒥᐦᐄᑯᑦ ᐊᓂᔫ ᑳ ᐧᐋᒐᑲᒥᑐᐧᐋᐱᔭᒡ᙮

ᐁᑯᓐ, ᒌ ᐃᑌᔭᐦᑕᒻ, ᓇᒧᐃ ᒦᓐ ᓂᑲ ᐅᐦᒋ ᓂᑐᐧᐋᐸᒫᐤ ᐊᓐ ᑳ ᐧᐋᐧᐄᐦᑕᒨᑦ ᒉ ᐃᔑ ᒦᒋᓱᔮᓐ ᑲᔦ ᓇᒧᐃ ᒦᓐ ᓂᑲ ᐅᐦᒋ ᐃᑐᐦᑌᓐ ᓂᑐᐦᑯᐃᓂᑲᒥᑯᐦᒡ ᒉᒌ ᓂᑑ ᒋᔅᒉᔭᒥᑯᔮᓐ ᐁ ᓲᐧᐋᑲᒥᐦᐧᑫᔮᓐ᙮ ᐧᐄᔭ ᐊᓂᔫᐦ ᒉᐧᑳᔫᐦ ᒣᔦᔭᐦᑕᒥᐦᐄᑯᑦ ᐁᑯᓐ ᐊᓂᔫᐦ ᒉ ᐃᐦᑑᑕᐦᒃ ᐁᒄ ᑲᔦ ᒉ ᐴᓂᐦᑖᑦ ᐊᓂᔫᐦ ᒉᐧᑳᔫᐦ ᐁᑳ ᐧᐄᒋᐦᐄᑯᑦ᙮ ᐋᔥᑰ ᒥᒄ ᒋᑲ ᓂᑐᐧᐋᐸᒣᐤ ᓂᑐᐦᑯᐃᓐ, ᐁᐅᒄ ᑳᒌ ᐃᐦᑎᑦ ᒫᓐ ᐊᓂᑌ ᐯᒋ ᒥᒄ ᐁᒌ ᓂᑑ ᒋᔅᒉᔭᒫᑲᓅᑦ ᒫᓐᐦ᙮ ᓇᒧᐃ ᒥᒄ ᒋᑲ ᐅᐦᒋ ᐃᑐᐦᑌᐤ ᐊᓂᔫ ᐅᐦᒋ ᐁ ᓲᐧᐋᑲᒥᐦᐧᑫᑦ ᐧᐄᔖᒫᑲᓅᑌ᙮

ça de travers; et elle devrait manger plus de ci et ça; et bla bla bla bla bla bla.

doing this wrong and that wrong and she should eat more of this and less of that and blah blah blah blah blah blah blah.

Elle rentra à pied de la clinique et réfléchit à tout ça.

She walked home from the clinic and thought about it.

Vraiment, ce n'était que négativité et confusion et ça n'aidait pas du tout. Elle ne voulait pas que quelqu'un d'autre lui dise ce qu'elle faisait de travers ou quoi manger ou qu'elle était trop grosse - elle avait eu assez de tout ça avec ce bon vieux Monsieur Les-yeux-bleus.

Really, it was just all negativity and confusion and it wasn't helping at all. She didn't want someone else telling her what she was doing wrong or what to eat or that she was too fat – she'd had enough of all that with ol' Blue Eyes.

*C'est fini,* se dit-elle, *plus de nutritionniste, plus de rendez-vous concernant mon diabète*. Elle continuerait à faire ce qui l'aidait à se sentir mieux et à ne pas faire ce qui la faisait se sentir mal. Elle irait voir le médecin de temps en temps, comme elle l'avait toujours fait, pour des examens généraux. Toutefois, elle ne le ferait plus pour des rendez-vous concernant le diabète.

*That's it,* she thought, *No more nutritionist, no more diabetes appointments.* She would keep on doing stuff that made her feel better and would keep on not doing stuff that made her feel worse. She'd check in with the doctor every now and again, like she always had, for general check-ups. But not for diabetes appointments.

ᒌᐦ ᐧᐋᐦᒌᔨᑰ ᐋᑳ ᐄᑐᐦᑖᑦ ᓂᑐᐦᑯᔨᓂᑭᒥᑯᐦᒡ᙮ ᓂᒧᐃ ᐹᔨᑯᐲᓯᒻ ᑭᑎ ᐃᐦᑖᐤ ᒑ ᒌᐦ ᒋᐱᐦᒌᑦ ᐧᐄ ᐊᓂᔮ᙮ ᒋᑭ ᒌᐦ ᐃᐦᑐᑎᒻ ᒥᒄ ᐹᔨᑯᒌᔑᑳᐤᐦ᙮

ᒥᒄ ᒫᒃ ᐹᔨᑯᓂᔨᐤ ᒑᐧᑳᔨᐤ ᒐ ᐧᐄᐦ ᓈᑭᑎᐧᐋᔨᐦᑎᐦᒃ᙮ ᐋᔪᐧᐃᒄ ᐊᓂᔮ ᓈᔥᒡ ᑳ ᒥᐧᔮᔨᐦᑎᐦᒃ ᑯᑫᐃᓐ᙮ ᒉᓂᕓᕐ ᐋᔥᒄ ᐋᔑᑯᒥᒌᔑᑳᐤᐦ ᒌᐦ ᐄᐦᑐᑎᒻ ᐊᓂᔮ ᑭᔮᐦ ᓂᒧᐃ ᐅᐦᒋ ᒫᔥᑎᓈᐦᐆ ᐧᐋᐦ ᐴᓂᐦᑖᐧᑳ᙮ ᓂᒥᔮᔨᐤ ᑭᔨᐧᐹ ᐋᐦ ᑯᔥᑎᐦᒃ ᒐ ᐃᐦᑎᒃ ᐃᔅᑯᑎᒃ ᐴᓂᐦᑖᒑ = ᓂᒧᐃ ᐧᐄ ᐊᓂᔮ ᐅᐦᒋ ᑯᔥᑎᒻ = ᒥᒄ ᓈᔥᒡ ᐋᐦ ᒌᐦ ᒥᔪᒥᒋᐦᐅᑦ ᐃᔮᐱᒋᐦᑖᒡᐦ᙮ ᐋᑦ ᒫᒃ ᐊᓂᔮ ᔒᔥ ᓈᔥᒡ ᓈᐅᔥ ᐋᐦ ᒌᐦ ᐋᐱᒋᐦᑖᑦ ᐊᔮᐱᒡ ᓈᐦᐋᐤ ᐊᐧᑳᔥᐱᔑ ᒥᔪᒥᒋᐦᐅᑦ ᐃᔮᐱᒋᔥᑖᒡᐦ᙮ ᐊᓂᔮ ᒫᒃ ᑳ ᒋᔥᒌᑦ ᐋᐦ ᐱᐹᒧᐦᑖᑦ ᑭᔮᐦ ᐋᐦ ᒌᐦ ᐴᓂᐦᑖᑦ ᐊᓂᔮ ᓂᑎᐧᐄ ᐋᐦ ᐄᔑᓈᑯᓂᔨᒡ ᒑᐧᑳᔨᐤ ᐋᐦ ᒦᒋᑦ ᑭᔮᐦ ᐋᐦ ᒌᐦ ᐴᓃᑦ ᐋᐦ ᒥᓂᐦᐧᑳᑦ, ᐊᔮᐱᒡ ᓈᐦᐋᐤ ᑳ ᐄᔥᐱᔑ ᒥᔪᒥᒋᐦᐅᑦ ᐋᐦ ᐋᐱᒋᔥᑖᑦ ᐊᓂᔮ ᑯᑫᐃᓂᔨᐤ᙮ ᐋᑯᑖᐦ ᑳ ᐄᑖᔨᐦᑎᐦᒃ ᐊᑎᑎᐤ ᒑ ᒥᔪᒥᒋᐦᐅᑯᐱᓈ ᑯᑫᐃᓐ ᐋᐦ ᐋᐱᒋᔥᑖᑦ ᐄᔑᐱᔑᐧᐄ ᐋᑳ ᓈᔥᑎᔨᒡ ᒑᐧᑳᔨᐤ ᐋᐱᒋᔥᑖᑦ᙮

ᐊᔮᐱᒡ ᒫᒃ, ᑳ ᐄᑖᔨᐦᑎᐦᒃ ᒑ ᑯᒋᔥᑖᑦ ᐋᑳ ᒑ ᐋᐱᒋᔥᑖᑦ ᐹᔨᑯᐲᓯᒻ ᐄᔥᐱᔥ᙮ ᐱᔑᓈ ᐊᑎᑎᐤ ᒋᐱᐦ ᒧᔪᐦᐧᑳᒨ᙮ ᒌᐦ ᒥᔮᔨᐦᑎᒥᔨᐤᐦ ᑭᔮᐦ ᐅᑎᐧᐋᔑᔒᒻᐦ ᐋᐦ ᑯᒋᔥᑖᑦ᙮ ᐋᐦ ᐧᐋᐱᒫᑯᑦ ᐋᑦ ᐋᑳ ᓈᔥᒡ ᒌᐦ ᐧᐋᒋᔨᑯᑦ ᒥᒄ ᒫᒃ ᒌᐦ ᒥᔮᐧᔮᔨᐦᒥᔨᐤᐦ ᓈᓈᓂᒌᒻ ᓰᐦᒃ ᐋᐦ ᑯᒋᔥᑖᑦ᙮

ᓇᒧᐃ ᓂᑲ ᐅᐦᒋ ᐋᔨᒥᐦᐄᑰᓐ ᒉᒌ ᐴᓂᔮᓐ ᓂᑐᐦᑯᐃᓂᑲᒥᑯᐦᒡ ᐁ ᐃᑐᐦᑌᔮᓐ ᒌ ᐃᑌᔨᐦᑕᒻ᙮ ᓇᒧᐃ ᒉᒋᒻ ᐯᔭᒄ ᐲᓯᒻ ᓵᔅ ᓇᒧᐃ ᓂᑲ ᐅᐦᒋ ᐃᑌᔨᐦᑌᓐ ᒉᒌ ᐄᑐᐦᑌᔮᓐ ᐊᓂᑌ᙮ ᒉᒋᒻ ᐊᓅᐦᒌᔥ ᓵᔅ ᓂᑲᒌ ᐴᓂᔨᓐ ᐊᓂᑌ ᐁ ᐄᑐᐦᑌᔮ ᒌ ᐄᑌᔨᐦᑕᒻ᙮

ᒫᐦᒋᔥᑕᐃ ᐯᔭᒄ ᑫᐧᑳᔫ ᒌ ᐃᐦᑕᑯᓂᔫ ᐁ ᒧᑯᔥᑳᒋᐦᑖᐤ ᑫᐧᐄ ᐴᓂᐦᑖᑦ᙮ ᐁᔅᒄ ᓈᔅᒡ ᑖᐧᐯ ᒌ ᒥᔐᔨᐦᑕᒻ ᐁ ᐃᐦᑑᑕᐦᒃ᙮ ᒉᔑᑯᒻ ᒌᔑᑳᐤᐦ ᒌ ᐃᐦᑑᑕᒻ ᑲᔐ ᓇᒧᐃ ᐅᐦᒋ ᒉᔅᑎᓈᓅ ᐧᐄᔅᑲᒡ ᑫᐧᐄ ᐴᓂᐦᑖᐧᑫ᙮ ᓇᒧᐃ ᑮᐸ ᐧᐄ ᐁ ᓴᒋᓯᑦ ᑖᓐ ᑫ ᐃᔅᐸᔨᑦ ᓯᔅᒋᑰᑦ ᐧᐄᐦ ᐴᓂᐦᑖᑌ = ᓇᒧᐃ ᐅᐦᒋ ᓴᒋᐦᐄᑰ ᐧᐁᔅ ᒌ ᒥᔐᔨᐦᑖᑯᓐ ᐁ ᐋᐸᒋᐦᑖᑦ ᐊᐧᐁᓐ ᑳ ᐧᐋᐹᔨᒡ ᒪᒋᓂᑐᐦᑯᐃᓂᔫ, ᒌ ᐃᑌᔨᐦᑕᒻ᙮ ᒥᐦᑫᑐ ᐱᐳᓐᐦ ᒌ ᐋᐸᒋᐦᑖᐤ ᐅᔫ ᒪᒋᓂᑐᐦᑯᐃᓂᔫ ᐁᔅᒄ ᒫᒃ ᓈᔅᒡ ᒥᔐᔨᐦᑖᑯᓐ ᐁ ᐃᐦᑑᑖᑲᓅᐦᒡ ᒌ ᐃᑌᔨᐦᑕᒻ᙮ ᑳᐦ ᒋᐦᒋᐸᔨᐦᑖᑦ ᒫᓐᐦ ᐁ ᐱᒧᐦᑌᑦ ᑲᔐ ᑯᐃᔅᒄ ᐁ ᐃᔑ ᒦᒋᓱᑦ ᑲᔐ ᐁ ᐴᓃᑦ ᐁ ᒥᓂᐦᐧᑫᑦ ᒌ ᒨᔑᐦᑖᐤ ᑖᐧᐯ ᐧᐁᑖᒡ ᐁ ᒥᔫᒪᐦᒋᐦᐆᑦ᙮ ᒥᒄ ᒫᒃ ᒌ ᐃᑌᔨᐦᑕᒻ ᐅᔥᑌ ᐁ ᒥᔫᒪᐦᒋᐦᐆᑦ ᐁ ᐅᑎᓇᐦᒃ ᑳ ᐧᐋᐹᔨᒡ ᒪᒋᓂᑐᐦᑯᐃᓂᔫ ᐃᔥᐱᔥ ᐧᐄ ᑖᓐ ᒋᐹ ᐃᑕᒪᐦᒋᐦᐆ ᐴᓂᐦᑖᑦ ᐊᓂᔫᐦ ᑯᑕᒃ ᑫᐧᑳᔫᐦ᙮

ᒌ ᑯᒋᐦᑖᔮᓐ ᑮᐹ ᐁᔫᐧᐁᐦᒡ ᐯᔭᑯᐲᓯᒻ, ᒌ ᐃᑌᔨᐦᑕᒻ᙮ ᓇᓂᑑ ᑮᐹ ᒋᐹ ᐧᐄᒋᐦᐄᑰ ᒉᒌ ᒥᔫᐦᐧᑳᒧᑦ᙮ ᑲᔐ ᒫᒃ ᐅᑕᐧᐋᔒᒻ ᒋᐹ ᒥᔐᔨᐦᑕᒥᔫᐦ ᐧᐋᐸᒥᑯᑦ ᐁ ᑯᒋᐦᑖᑦ ᒉᒌ ᐧᐄᒋᐦᐄᓱᑦ᙮ ᐧᐋᐸᒥᑯᑦ ᐁᑳ ᑲᔅᒋᐦᐅᑦ ᓃᔥᑕᒻ ᑫᒃ ᒫᒃ ᐧᐁᑖᒡ ᐊᑎ ᓇᑲᔭᒥᐦᑖᑦ᙮

Cesser d'aller à la clinique était facile. Elle n'allait pas avoir besoin d'un mois pour se sevrer de ça. Elle pouvait le faire en un jour.

Quitting the clinic was easy. She wasn't gonna need a month to wean herself off of that. She could do it in one day.

Elle n'avait plus qu'une habitude dont prendre le contrôle. La belle, belle poudre. Jennifer en prenait encore tous les jours et elle n'était pas sûre de vouloir arrêter. Non pas parce qu'elle craignait le sevrage – ce n'était pas le cas –, mais parce que la cocaïne lui procurait une sensation incroyable. Même après toutes ces années, c'était incroyable. Lorsqu'elle avait commencé à marcher et qu'elle avait cessé de consommer de la malbouffe puis de boire, elle avait toujours fini par se sentir mieux. Toutefois, elle était presque sûre qu'elle se sentait beaucoup mieux défoncée à la cocaïne qu'elle ne se sentirait jamais si elle était *clean*.

There was just one more habit to get under control. Beautiful, beautiful blow. Jennifer was still using every day and she wasn't entirely sure she wanted to quit. Not because she feared withdrawal – she didn't – but because cocaine felt amazing. Even after all these years it felt amazing. When she had started walking and had stopped junk food and then drinking, she had always eventually felt better for it. But she was pretty sure that she felt a whole lot better high on blow than she ever would feel if she were clean.

Elle pourrait quand même essayer pendant un mois. Elle dormirait probablement mieux. Ce serait bien aussi pour les enfants, de la voir essayer. De la voir ne pas être bonne dans un domaine, mais essayer de s'améliorer.

Still, she could try it for a month. She'd probably sleep better. It'd be good for the kids, too, to see her try. To see her not be good at something and then try to get better at it.

ᑮᔮᐦ ᒫᒃ ᐧᑳᐧᔖᓐ ᐋᔮᐱᒡ ᒋᑭ ᒌᐦ ᐋᐱᒋᔥᑖᐤ ᑯᑫᐃᓂᔨᐤ ᓈᔥᒡ ᒥᒄ ᓂᔮᓂᑯᑑᓐᐦ᙮

ᐊᓂᔮᐦ ᓃᔥᑎᒻ ᓃᔓᒌᔑᑳᐤᐦ ᓈᔥᒡ ᐋᐦ ᒌᐦ ᒫᑯᐦᐄᑯᑦ᙮ ᓂᒧᐃ ᒥᒄ ᑳ ᐄᔥᐱᔑ ᒫᑯᐦᐄᑯᑦ ᑳ ᐴᓂᐦᑖᑦ ᓂᑎᐧᐄ ᒑᐧᑳᔨᐤ ᐋᐦ ᒦᒋᑦ, ᒥᒄ ᒫᒃ ᐋᔮᐱᒡ ᓈᔥᒡ ᒌᐦ ᒫᑯᐦᐄᑰ᙮ ᒉᓂᔕᕐ ᓂᒥ ᓈᔥᒡ ᐅᐦᒋ ᐧᐄᐦ ᐃᔮᐱᑖᔨᐦᑎᒻ᙮ ᒌᐦ ᐋᐱᑎᓰᐤ ᐋᔮᐱᒡ ᑮᔮᐦ ᒌᐦ ᑭᓂᐧᐋᔨᒫᐤ ᐅᑎᐧᐋᔑᔒᒻᐦ ᑮᔮᐦ ᒌᐦ ᐧᐋᐧᐄᒑᐧᐋᐤ ᐅᐧᐄᒑᐧᐋᑭᓐᐦ, ᐋᑦ ᒫᒃ ᐊᓂᔮ ᐋᑎ ᐃᔨᐦᑎᒃ ᐋᔮᐱᒡ ᒌᐦ ᒋᔅᒋᓰᑎᑎᒻ ᑯᑫᐃᓐ ᑮᔮᐦ ᐊᓂᔮ ᑳ ᐄᑎᒥᒋᐦᐅᑦ ᐃᔅᑯᑎᒃ ᐋᔅᑯᑖᒧᑎᑎᒃᐦ, ᑮᔮᐦ ᒨᔮᒻ ᒥᓯᐧᐋ ᒑᐧᑳᔨᐤ ᒐ ᒥᔪᐱᔨᔨᒡ᙮ ᐊᓂᔮ ᓃᔥᑎᒻ ᑳ ᑎᐧᐃᔥᑖᔨᒡ ᓈᔥᒡ ᐋᐦ ᒌᐦ ᑭᒋᔑᐧᐋᐦᐄᑯᑦ ᒥᓯᐧᐋ ᒑᐧᑳᔨᐤ ᑮᔮᐦ ᒋᔥᒋᑯᒡ ᑳ ᒌ ᐃᐦᑎᒃ ᒋᔥᒋᑯᒡ ᐋᐦ ᐄᔑ ᑭᒋᓯᐧᐋᓯᑦ᙮

ᓂᔮᓂᑯᑑᓐᐦ ᐊᓂᑖᐦ ᐧᐋᑖᑯᔑᔨᒡᐦ, ᑳ ᒌ ᐲᐦᐧᑖᑎᑎᒃᐦ ᐋᑯᑎᐦ ᐊᐱᔒᔥ ᑳ ᐧᐄᒋᐦᐄᑯᑦ᙮ ᓂᒥ ᓈᔥᒡ ᐅᐦᒋ ᒋᔑᐱᔨᔨᐤ ᐅᑖᐃᐦ ᑮᔮᐦ ᓂᒥ ᓈᔥᒡ ᐅᐦᒋ ᒦᒋᓈᑯᓂᔨᐤᐦ ᐅᔥᒌᔑᒄᐦ᙮

ᒑᒃ ᒦᓐ ᐹᑎᒫᐦ, ᑳ ᐄᔅᑯᑖᒥᑎᐦᒃ ᒦᓐ ᑯᑫᐃᓐ᙮ ᓇᔥᒡ ᐋᐦ ᒌᐦ ᑯᔥᐧᑳᔨᐦᑎᐦᒃ ᐋᑳ ᓈᔥᒡ ᒧᔑᐦᑖᑦ ᐊᓂᔮ ᑳ ᒌ ᐃᐦᑐᑖᑯᑦ ᒫᓐᐦ᙮ ᐋᔮᐱᒡ ᑭᔨᐧᐹ ᑳ ᒌ ᒋᔅᒋᓰᑎᑎᒃᐦ = ᒥᒄ ᒫᒃ ᒌᐦ ᒋᔅᒑᔨᐦᑎᒻ ᐋᑳ ᑖᐧᐹᐦ ᓂᑎᐧᐋᔨᐦᑎᐦᒃ᙮ ᒌᐦ ᒋᔅᒑᔨᐦᑎᒻ ᐋᑳ ᓈᔥᑎᔨᒡ ᐧᐄᒋᐦᐄᑯᑦ᙮ ᓈᔥᑎᔨᒡ ᓂᒥ ᐊᑎᑎᐤ

ᐁᒄ ᑳ ᐃᑌᔨᐦᑕᒃ ᒥᒄ ᓂᔮᓂᑯᑌᐦᒡ ᒉᒌ ᐋᐸᒋᐦᑖᑦ ᐊᓂᔫ ᒪᒋᓂᑐᐦᑯᐃᓂᔫ᙮

ᐅᔅᑲᒡ ᑳᐧᐄ ᐴᓂᐦᑖᑦ ᓈᔅᒡ ᑖᐧᐯ ᒌ ᐋᔨᒪᐦᐄᑰ᙮ ᓇᒧᐃ ᑮᐹ ᐅᐦᒋ ᐃᔥᐱᔥ ᐋᔨᒪᐦᐄᑰ ᑳ ᐃᔥᐱᔥ ᒌ ᐋᔨᒥᐦᐄᑯᑦ ᐅᔅᑲᒡ ᑳᐧᐄ ᐴᓂᐦᑖᑦ ᐁ ᓰᐅᒦᒋᓱᑦ ᑯᐃᔅᒄ ᐁᒌᐧᐄᔑ ᒦᒋᓱᑦ, ᔮᐸᒡ ᑮᐹ ᓄᐧᐊᒡ ᐋᐃᒪᓐ ᒌ ᐄᑌᔨᐦᑕᒻ᙮ ᒌ ᐃᐦᑑᑕᒻ ᐊᓂᔫᐦ ᒉᐧᑳᔫᐦ ᒋᐹ ᐃᐦᑑᑕᒻ ᒣᔑᑯᒻ ᒌᔑᑳᐤᐦ᙮ ᒌ ᓂᑑ ᐋᐸᑎᓰ ᑲᔦ ᒌ ᓇᓈᑲᑕᐧᐁᔨᒣᐤ ᐅᑕᐧᐋᔒᒻ ᑲᔦ ᐅᐧᐄᒉᐧᐋᑲᓐᐦ ᒌ ᐧᐋᐸᒣᐤ ᐋᔥᑰ, ᒥᒄ ᒫᒃ ᔮᐸᒡ ᐋᔥᑰ ᒌ ᑲᐧᑫᑌᔨᐦᑕᒻ ᒉᒌ ᐅᑎᓇᐦᒃ ᐊᓂᔫ ᑳ ᐧᐋᐹᔨᒡ ᒪᒋᓂᑎᐦᑯᐃᓂᔫ, ᐁ ᒋᔅᑫᔨᐦᑕᒃ ᑫ ᐃᐦᑑᑖᑯᑦ ᒥᒄ ᐧᐁᐃᐱᔅᒌᔥ ᐁᑳ ᒥᒍᓐ ᑫ ᐅᐦᒋ ᒥᑯᔥᑳᑌᔨᐦᑕᒥᐦᐄᑯᑦ ᑫᐧᑳᔫ᙮ ᐊᓂᔫ ᒫᒃ ᓃᔥᑕᒻ ᐯᔮᒄ ᑑᔥᑌᐤ ᐅᔥᑌᔒᔥ ᒫᒃ ᐁᑳ ᐅᐦᒋ ᐅᑎᓇᐦᒃ ᑫᐧᑳᔫ ᓈᔅᒡ ᒨᔥ ᒌᐧᐃ ᒋᔥᑳᔦᔨᐦᑕᒻ ᒌ ᐃᑌᔨᐦᑖᑯᓰ ᐁᑳ ᓈᔥᒡ ᐋᐸᑌᔨᐦᑖᑯᓂᔨᒡ ᑫᐧᑳᔫ ᐁᒌ ᐅᐦᒋ ᒋᔑᐧᐋᓯᑦ᙮

ᓂᔮᓂᑯᑌᐦᒡ ᐁ ᐅᑖᑯᔑᔨᒡ, ᒌ ᐲᐦᐧᑖᐤ ᒪᒋᒋᔥᑌᒫᐤᐦ ᒉᒌ ᐅᐦᒋ ᒋᔮᒣᔨᒧᑦ᙮ ᐅᔫ ᐁ ᐃᐦᑎᑦ ᓇᒧᐃ ᐅᐦᒋ ᐃᔥᐱᔥ ᒋᔑᐸᐦᑖᒪᑲᓂᔫ ᐅᑌᐦᐄ ᑲᔦ ᓇᒧᐃ ᐅᐦᒋ ᒪᒋᑯᐦᑎᓂᔫᐦ ᐅᔅᒌᔑᒄᐦ᙮

ᐹᑎᒫᔒᔥ ᒫᒃ, ᒦᓐ ᒌ ᐃᔥᐸᑖᐦᑕᒻ ᐊᓂᔫ ᑳ ᐧᐋᐹᔨᒡ ᒪᒋᓂᑐᐦᑯᐃᓂᔫ᙮ ᒌ ᑯᔥᐧᑫᔨᐦᑕᒻ ᒫᒃ ᐁᑳ ᐅᐦᒋ ᐧᐄ ᐋᐦᐸᑲᐦᐄᑯᑦ᙮ ᔮᐸᒡ ᒫᒃ ᓂᔮᓂᑯᑌᐦᒡ ᒌ ᓂᑐᐧᐁᔨᐦᑕᒻ = ᐧᐁᔥ ᑳ ᐧᐋᐹᔨᒡ ᒪᒋᓂᑐᐦᑯᐃᓂᔫ ᐊᓂᔫ = ᒥᒄ ᒫᒃ ᓇᒧᐃ ᑖᐧᐯ ᐅᐦᒋ ᓂᑐᐧᐁᔨᐦᑕᒡ᙮ ᓇᒧᐃ ᐅᐦᒋ ᓂᑐᐧᐁᔨᐦᑕᒻ

Et peut-être qu'elle pourrait encore se faire une ligne toutes les quelques semaines environ.

Les deux premiers jours la virent subir des envies intenses. Pas aussi fortes que ses envies de sucre quand elle avait arrêté la malbouffe, mais quand même assez fortes. Jennifer fit le nécessaire. Elle alla au travail, s'occupa de ses enfants et passa du temps avec ses amis, mais, pendant tout ce temps, elle pensait à sniffer des lignes de poudre blanche et à cette effervescence électrique quand elle atteignait votre cerveau, quand vous saviez que pendant quelques minutes tout irait bien. Et, pendant la première semaine environ, elle était tellement à cran que la moindre petite chose la mettait en colère.

Parfois, le soir, elle fumait un peu d'herbe pour se détendre. Ça faisait l'affaire et n'affolait pas son cœur ni faisait paraître ses yeux étranges.

Après quelques semaines, elle sniffa une ligne de cocaïne. Étonnamment, la défonce ne fut pas aussi bien que ça. Elle en avait toujours envie, bien sûr – c'était de la cocaïne –, cependant elle n'en avait pas vraiment besoin. Ça ne valait pas ce

And maybe she could still do a line every few weeks or so.

The first couple of days brought some intense cravings. Not as bad as the sugar cravings had been when she cut out junk food, but still, pretty bad. Jennifer went through the motions. She went to work and looked after her kids and hung out with her friends, but, through it all, she thought about sniffing back lines of white powder and that electric buzz when it hit your brain, when you knew that for a few minutes everything would be all right. And for the first week or so, she was so cranky that any little thing would set her off.

Sometimes, in the evenings, she smoked a bit of weed to take the edge off. It did the trick and didn't make her heart race nor her eyes look weird.

After a few weeks, she snorted a line of blow. Surprisingly, the high wasn't really all that great. She still craved it, of course – it was cocaine – but she didn't really need it. It wasn't worth what it took out of her. She was done with it. Without

ᐅᐦᒋ ᐃᔮᐱᑖᔨᐦᑎᒻ᙮ ᓂᒧᐃ ᐅᐦᒋ ᐃᔨᑐᐦᑖᐤ ᐧᐄᔮᔥᑖᐦ ᒑ ᒌᐦ ᐧᐄᒋᐦᐋᑭᓂᐧᐃᑦ ᐅᐦᒋ ᐊᓂᔮ ᒑᐧᑳᔨᐤ ᑳ ᐋᑎ ᐃᔨᔮᐱᒋᐦᑖᑦ ᑭᔮᐦ ᓂᒥ ᐧᐋᐧᐋᒡ ᐅᐦᒋ ᐊᔨᒥᐦᐋᐤ ᒋᔖᔨᔨᐤᐦ, ᐧᐄᔨ ᒥᒄ ᒌᐦ ᐃᐦᑐᑎᒻ ᐋᑳ ᒑ ᐃᔮᐱᑖᔨᐦᑎᐦᒃ ᐊᓂᔮ ᑯᑫᐃᓂᔨᐤ᙮

ᐊᓂᔮ ᒫᒃ ᑳ ᐴᓃᑭᐦᒃ ᑯᑫᐃᓐ ᐊᑎᑎᐤ ᒌᐦ ᐧᐋᐦᒌᔨᑰ ᑳ ᐃᐦᑎᒃ ᑳ ᐧᐄᐦ ᐴᓂᐦᑖᑦ ᓂᑎᐧᐄ ᒑᐧᑳᔨᐤ ᐋᐦ ᒦᒋᑦ᙮

ᒑᒃ ᑳ ᒥᐢᑭᐦᒃ ᑫᓂᔕᐠ ᐋᐱᑎᓰᐧᐄᓂᔨᐤ᙮ ᓂᒥ ᓈᔥᒡ ᐅᐦᒋ ᒫᑯᐦᐄᑯᐧᐃᒡ ᒑᐧᑳᔨᐤ ᐅᐦᒋ ᔓᐧᐃᔮᓐᐦ ᐊᓂᑖᐦ ᐧᐄᒋᐦᐧᐋᐦᒡ᙮ ᓂᒥ ᐅᐦᒋ ᐴᓃᐤ ᑭᔮᐦ ᐋᐦ ᐱᐹᒥᐦᑖᑦ ᑭᔮᐦ ᐋᐦ ᒫᒥᑐᓈᔨᐦᑎᐦᒃ᙮

ᒑᑳᑦ ᒫᒃ ᒨᔥ ᑳ ᐄᑎᒥᐦᐅᑦ ᒨᔮᒻ ᐋᐦ ᐧᐄᐦ ᐹᑯᒧᑦ᙮ ᐊᓅᐦᒡ ᒫᒃ ᐊᑎᑎᐤ ᓈᔥᒡ ᒌᐦ ᒥᔨᐦᒥᐦᒋᐦᐆ, ᒥᒄ ᒫᒃ ᐋᔥᒄ ᐊᔮᐱᒡ ᓂᒥ ᐅᐦᒋ ᐃᐦᑎᐤ ᐊᓂᑖᐦ ᒋᔥᒋᐧᐋ ᒑ ᒌᐦ ᒥᔨᒥᐦᒋᐦᐅᑦ ᑮᔮᐦ ᓈᔥᒡ ᐋᑳ ᐅᐦᒋ ᓵᐹᑭᒥᔨᒡ ᐅᒥᐦᒄ = ᐋᑯᐦ ᑳ ᒥᔮᑭᓂᐧᐃᑦ ᓂᑐᐦᑯᔨᓐᐦ ᒑ ᐋᐱᒋᐦᑖᑦ ᒥᒄ ᒫᒃ ᓈᔥᒡ ᐋᐦ ᒌᐦ ᒋᐱᑭᐦᒑᐦᐅᑯᑦ᙮ ᐊᓂᑖᐦ ᒫᒃ ᐋᐦ ᐋᐱᑎᓰᑦ ᑫᓂᔕᐠ, ᒫᐧᑳᒡ ᐋᐦ ᐃᔮᔨᒧᑎᒥᔨᒡᐦ ᐊᓂᔮᐦ ᐅᐧᐄᒑᐱᑎᓯᒪᑭᓐᐦ ᐹᑎᒫᐦ ᒑ ᒥᓂᐦᐧᑳᔨᒡᐦ ᑮᔮᐦ ᐧᐃᔨᐧᐄᑎᒥᐦᒡ ᒑ ᐱᒥᓂᐧᐋᔨᒡᐦ ᐴᓇᐱᑎᓯᔨᒥᐦᐋ, ᐧᐄᔨ ᑫᓂᔕᐠ ᒥᒄ ᒦᓯᐅᑭᒥᑯᔨᐤ ᐋᔦᐧᐃᒄ ᑳ ᒋᐢᒋᓰᑎᑎᐦᒃ᙮ ᐊᓂᑖᐦ ᒫᒃ ᐹᐹᒧᐦᑖᒡᐦ ᐊᑎᑎᐤ ᒌᐦ ᒋᐢᒋᓰᑎᑎᒻ: ᒋᑭ ᒥᔦᐱᔨᐧᐋ ᐄᑐᐦᑖᔮᓈ ᒦᓐ ᒦᓯᐅᑭᒥᑯᐦᒡ,

ᒦᓐ ᑫᒌ ᐃᐦᔫᑖᑯᑦ ᑫᒌ ᐧᐊᓂᐦᑖᑦ ᑖᓐ ᑳ ᐃᔑ ᐊᔮᑦ ᐅᐱᒫᑎᓰᐧᐃᓂᐦᒡ᙮ ᔮᐢ ᒋᐦᒋᐧᐁ ᓂᑲ ᐴᓂᐦᑖᓐ ᒌ ᐃᑌᔨᐦᑕᒻ᙮ ᐋᑦ ᐁᑳ ᐅᐦᒋ ᐃᐦᑖᑦ ᐊᓂᑌ ᐧᐁᐦᒋ ᐧᐄᒋᐦᐋᑲᓅᐧᑖᐤ ᐊᐧᐁᓂᒌ, ᒫᒃ ᐊᓂᑌ ᓀᔥᑑᐱᐧᑖᐤ ᒫᓐ ᐊᐧᐁᓂᒌ ᒥᓂᐦᐧᑫᐧᐃᓂᔫ ᒫᒃ ᒪᒋᓂᑐᐦᑯᐃᓐᐦ ᐁᐧᐄ ᐃᐢᐸᔑᐦᐄᑯᐧᑖᐤ ᓇᒧᐃ ᑲᔦ ᐅᐦᒋ ᐊᔨᒥᐦᐁᐤ ᐁ ᒋᔒᓈᔨᒡ ᐊᐧᐁᔫ ᑫᒌ ᐧᐄᒋᐦᐄᑯᑦ ᔮᐸᒡ ᒌ ᐃᐦᑑᑕᒻ ᐁᑳ ᑫᒌ ᐱᐢᑫᔨᐦᑕᐦᒃ ᐊᓂᔫ ᒪᒋᓂᑐᐦᑯᐃᓂᔫ᙮

ᐁᑎᑑ ᒌ ᐧᐁᐦᒋᐦᐄᑯ ᐅᔫ ᐁ ᐴᓂᐦᑖᑦ ᐃᔥᐱᔥ ᐧᐄ ᒦᒋᒥᔫ ᐁᑳ ᒥᔫᐢᑲᑫᔨᒡ᙮ ᒌ ᐃᔑᓈᑯᓂᔫ ᒫᒃ ᑫᒌ ᒫᒥᑐᓀᔨᐦᑕᐦᒃ ᐅᔫ᙮

ᑫᒃ ᒫᒃ ᒌ ᐃᔑᓈᑯᓂᔫ ᑫᒌ ᐊᔮᑦ ᐋᐸᑎᓯᐧᐃᓂᔫ ᑫᓂᔕᐠ᙮ ᒌ ᒥᔫᐸᔫᒡ ᐊᓂᑕ ᐁ ᐯᔭᑯᑌᐅᓰᐧᑖᐤ ᔔᓕᔮᔫ ᐁ ᐊᔮᐧᑖᐤ᙮ ᐅᒄ ᒋᓯᓀ ᑳ ᐃᐦᑎᑦ ᐁ ᐱᒧᐦᑌᑦ ᑲᔦ ᐁ ᒫᒥᑐᓀᔨᐦᑕᒃ᙮

ᒌ ᒫᒥᑐᓀᔨᐦᑕᒥᐦᐄᑰ ᐅᔓ ᑫ ᐃᐢᐸᔨᑦ ᒦᓰᐅᑲᒥᑯᐦᒡ ᐊᐱᑌ᙮ ᐋᒥᓀ ᑮᐹ ᒌ ᐃᑕᒪᐦᒋᐦᐆ ᐁᑯ, ᒥᒄ ᒫᒃ ᐁᐢᑯ ᓇᒧᐃ ᐅᐦᒋ ᒥᔫᐸᔫ ᐧᐃᔮᐦᒡ ᐊᓂᔫ ᐅᐦᒋ ᐁᒌ ᐧᑫᔥᑎᓇᐦᒃ ᑖᓐ ᑳ ᐄᑖᑎᓰᑦ = ᒌ ᓂᑐᐧᐁᔨᐦᑖᑯᓂᔫ ᑫᒌ ᐅᑎᓇᐦᒃ ᓂᑐᐦᑯᐃᓐᐦ ᑫᒌ ᓵᐸᒪᐦᒋᐦᐅᑦ ᒥᒄ ᒫᒃ ᒌ ᒋᐸᑲᐦᑫᐦᐆᑰ ᐊᓂᔫᐦ᙮ ᐊᓂᑌ ᔮᐸᑎᓯᑦ, ᐊᓂᔫᐦ ᐧᐃᔮᐸᑎᓰᒪᑦ ᒌ ᓂᑑ ᒥᓂᐦᐧᑫᔫᐦ ᑲᔦ ᑯᑕᒃ ᒌ ᓂᑑ ᒦᒋᓯᔫᐦ ᒫᓐᐦ ᐁᑯ ᐧᐃ ᑫᓂᔕᐠ ᒌ ᒫᒥᑐᓀᔨᐦᑕᒥᐦᐄᑯ ᑫ ᒥᔫᐧᐁᐱᓇᒥᐧᑫ ᑫᐧᑳᔫ ᒦᓰᐅᑲᒥᑯᐦᒡ ᐃᑐᐦᑌᑌ᙮ ᐯᐹᒧᐦᑌᒡ ᑲᔦ ᐁᐅᒄ ᐊᓂᔫ ᑳ ᒫᒥᑐᓀᔨᐦᑕᒥᐦᐄᑯᑦ, ᒦᓰᐅᑲᒥᑯᐦᒡ ᐃᑐᐦᑌᔮᓐ, ᒋᑲ ᒥᔫᐸᔫ ᑳᑲᔦ ᐁ ᒦᓰᔮᓐ᙮ ᒌ ᐄᑎᑰᑯᐸᓀ ᑮᐹ ᐅᓂᑐᐦᑯᐃᓂᒻ ᑫ ᐊᑎ ᒥᔫᐸᔨᑦ᙮ ᑖᐧᐯ ᒫᒃ᙮

que ça lui coûtait. Elle en avait fini avec elle. Sans réadaptation ni traitement, sans AA ni même en parler avec un aîné, elle avait réussi à maîtriser sa dépendance à la cocaïne.

rehab or treatment or AA or even talking with an Elder about it, she had brought her cocaine addiction under control.

Et cesser de prendre de la cocaïne avait été plus facile que de cesser de manger de la malbouffe. Ça faisait réfléchir aussi.

And stopping blow had been easier than stopping junk food. That was something to think about too.

Jennifer trouva finalement du travail. Financièrement, les choses se stabilisèrent à la maison. Elle continuait à marcher et à réfléchir.

Jennifer found work eventually. Financially things levelled out at home. She kept walking and thinking.

La moitié du temps, elle pensait à la salle de bain. Elle se sentait tellement mieux désormais, mais son corps s'habituait encore à tous les changements qu'elle avait effectué et il était devenu anémique – elle avait dû commencer à prendre des pilules de suppléments en fer et celles-ci l'avaient bouchée comme un drain plein de cheveux. Ainsi, au travail, quand tout le monde pensait à prendre un verre et à faire un barbecue après le travail, Jennifer pensait à la salle de bain. Et quand elle marchait autour de la piste, elle y pensait davantage : *Quand je vais aller à la salle*

Half the time, she was thinking about the toilet. She felt so much better now, but her body was still getting used to all the changes she had made and it had become anemic – she had had to go on iron pills and they plugged her up like a drain full of hair. So, at work, when everybody else was thinking about a drink and a barbeque after work, Jennifer was thinking about the toilet. And when she walked around the track, she thought about it more: *When I go to the toilet, is it actually gonna come?* The doctor said that would fix itself eventually. And it did.

ᐄᑖᔭᐦᑎᒻ᙮ ᑳ ᐄᑎᑯᑦ ᐧᐋᔥ ᐊᓂᔮᐦ ᓂᑐᐦᑯᔭᓐ ᓈᒃ ᐋᑳ ᐊᓂᔮ ᓈ ᐃᐦᑎᒃ᙮ ᑖᐧᐹᐦ ᒫᒃ ᐋᑯᑖᐦ ᑳ ᐄᔅᐱᔭᑦ᙮

ᑯᑎᒋᔭᐤ ᑭᔭᐧᐹ ᑳ ᒌ ᒫᒥᑐᓈᔭᐦᑎᒥᐦᐄᑯᑦ ᓈᐧᑳᔭᐤ, ᒫᐧᑳᒡ ᐊᓂᔮ ᐋᐦ ᐱᐹᒎᐦᑖᑦ᙮ ᐹᔭᒄ ᐊᓂᔮᐦ ᐧᐄᒋᔖᓂᔥᐦ, ᐊᓂᔮᐦ ᐹᔭᒄ ᐊᐧᐋᔭᐤᐦ ᓈᔥᒡ ᑳ ᒥᐧᔮᔭᒪᑦ, ᒌᐦ ᐃᔮᔨᐧᐃᐦᐄᑯᓯᔭᐤᐦ, ᐋᑯᑎᐦ ᒫᒃ ᒥᔥᑏᐦ ᓈᐧᑳᔭᐤ ᓂᒥ ᐅᐦᒋ ᒌᐦ ᓂᓯᑐᐦᑎᒻ᙮

ᐅᑎᐧᐋᔑᔒᒻᐦ ᑭᔮᐦ ᒌᐦ ᒋᔅᒋᓰᑎᑎᐧᐋᐤ᙮ "ᐅᐧᐋ ᓈᑳ, ᓂᐧᐃᒡ ᓂᒥ ᐧᐄᐦᑭᓐ ᐆ," ᑳ ᒌ ᐄᑎᑯᑦ ᒫᓐ ᐊᓂᔮᐦ ᐅᑯᓯᔅᐦ ᐋᔑᒫᒡᐦ ᓈᐧᑳᔭᐤ ᓈᔥᒡ ᓈ ᒥᔨᔥᑳᑯᔭᒡᐦ ᐅᔮᔭᐦᒡ, ᒥᑯ ᒫᒃ ᐋᔮᐱᒡ ᑳ ᒌᐦ ᒦᒋᔭᒡᐦ᙮ ᐊᑎᑎᐤ ᑯᐃᔅᑯ ᒌᐦ ᑭᓂᐧᐋᔭᒫᐤ ᐅᑎᐧᐋᔑᔒᒻᐦ ᑳ ᐄᔥᐱᔑ ᐊᑎᑎᐤ ᒥᔨᐱᒫᑎᓰᑦ᙮ ᓈᓈᓂᒌᒻ ᑭᔮᐦ ᐊᑎᑎᐤ ᒌᐦ ᒥᐧᔮᔭᒫᐤ ᐅᑎᐧᐋᔑᔒᒻᐦ ᑭᔮᐦ ᐊᑎᑎᐤ ᒌᐦ ᔒᐲᐧᐋᓯᐤ ᐅᐦᒋ ᐊᓂᔮᐦ ᐅᑎᐧᐋᔑᔒᒻᐦ᙮

ᐋᔥᒄ ᐋᔮᐱᒡ ᒌᐦ ᒋᔅᒋᓰᑎᑎᐧᐋᐤ ᓂᔮᓂᑯᑑᓐᐦ ᐊᓂᔮ ᑳ ᓂᑭᑎᑯᑦ ᐅᐧᐹᔭᒻᐦ᙮ ᑖᐹ ᐊᓂᑎᐦ ᐅᐦᒋ ᐃᐦᑖᔭᐤᐦ, ᐊᓂᑖᐦ ᑯᑎᒃ ᐃᐦᑖᐧᐃᓂᐦᒡ ᒌᐦ ᐄᔑ ᐋᐦᑐᒑᔭᐤᐦ ᐊᓂᑎᐦ ᑳ ᐃᐦᑖᔭᒡᐦ ᐊᓂᔮᐦ ᑯᑎᒃᐦ ᐅᑎᔅᐧᑳᒻᐦ ᑭᔮᐦ ᐅᑎᐧᐋᔑᔒᒻᐦ᙮ ᓈᓈᓂᒌᒻ ᒫᒃ ᒌᐦ ᐊᑎ ᐊᐱᔒᔑᐤ ᑫᓂᓭᑫ᙮ ᑳ ᒌ ᐄᑎᑯᑦ ᒫᓐ ᐊᐧᐋᔭᐤᐦ ᑳᐅᐦᑭᑎᐦᐄᓯᐧᑳ᙮ (ᓂᒧᐃ ᒫᒃ ᐅᔮ ᐅᐦᒋ ᐃᐦᑐᑎᒻ᙮) ᓈᔥᒡ ᐋᐦ ᒌᐦ ᑯᔥᑯᐦᐋᑦ ᑭᔮᐦ ᐊᓂᔮᐦ ᐅᓂᑐᐦᑯᔭᓂᒻᐦ ᑳ ᐲᐦᒋᒑᐧᐋᑦ

ᑯᑖᒃ ᑲᔦ ᑫᐧᑳᔩᐦ ᒌ ᒫᒥᑐᓀᔭᐦᑕᒥᐦᐄᑰ᙮ ᐧᐄᒌᓃᐦᑳᐧᐃᓐ ᓈᔅᒡ ᐁᒌ ᓵᒋᐦᐋᑦ, ᒌ ᐃᔥᐧᑳᓇᒥᔩᐦ ᐅᐱᒫᑎᓰᐧᐃᓂᔩ ᓇᒧᐃ ᒫᒃ ᐅᐦᒋ ᓂᓯᑐᐦᑕᒻ ᑫᐧᑳᔩ ᐧᐁᐦᒌ ᐃᔅᐸᔭᔭᒡ ᐅᔩ᙮

ᐅᑕᐧᐋᔒᒻᐦ ᑲᔦ ᒌ ᒫᒥᑐᓀᔭᒣᐤ᙮ "ᒫᒫ, ᒋᐧᐄ ᓂᐸᐦᐄᓐ ᐋ", ᒌ ᐄᑎᑰ ᐅᑯᔕ ᐯᒥᓄᐧᐁᒡ ᑫᐧᑳᔩ ᐁ ᒥᔩᔅᑳᑫᔭᒡ, ᒦᒄ ᑮᐹ ᔮᐸᒡ ᒌ ᒦᒋᔩᐦ᙮ ᐁᑎᑑ ᒌ ᒥᔩᔅᑲᐧᐃᔩ ᐁᒄ ᑳ ᒥᔩᐸᔭᓂᔭᒡ ᑫᒌ ᒥᔩᐦᑲᐧᐋᑦ ᐅᑕᐧᐋᔒᒻᐦ᙮ ᐁᑎᑑ ᒌ ᓵᒋᐦᐁᐤ ᐅᑕᐧᐋᔒᒻᐦ ᑲᔦ ᐁᑎᑑ ᒌ ᔒᐲᐧᐁᔒᔥᑕᐧᐁᐤ᙮

ᒌ ᒫᒥᑐᓀᔭᒣᐤ ᓂᔮᓂᑯᑌᒡ ᐊᓂᔩ ᓈᐯᐤ ᑳᒌ ᐧᐄᒋᒫᑦ᙮ ᓵᔅ ᑮᐹ ᓇᒧᐃ ᐅᐦᒋ ᐧᐄᑫᐅᑑᒡ, ᒌ ᐋᐦᒋᔥᑲᑕᒥᔩᐦ ᑲᔦ ᓵᔅ ᒌ ᐊᔮᐧᐁᐤ ᑯᑖᒃ ᐃᔅᐧᑫᐤᐦ ᑲᔦ ᒌ ᐅᑕᐧᐋᔑᒥᔩ᙮ ᒥᔅᑕᐦᐄ ᒌ ᐊᒎᐸᔩ ᑫᓂᓭᑫ, ᓇᒧᐃ ᐅᐦᒋ ᐃᔅᐱᒋᔥᑑ ᐊᓂᔩ ᑳᒌ ᐃᔅᐱᒋᔥᑎᑦ᙮ ᒋᐧᐄ ᑰᐦᑲᑎᐦᐄᓯᓐ ᐋ, ᒌ ᐄᑎᑰ ᒫᓐᐦ ᐊᐧᐁᔩᐦ᙮ ᓇᒧᐃ ᑮᐹ ᐅᐦᒋ ᐧᐄ ᑰᐦᑲᑎᐦᐄᓰ᙮ ᑲᔦ ᐅᓂᑐᐦᑯᐃᓂᒻ ᑳ ᓂᑑᐧᐋᐸᒫᑦ ᒌ ᑯᔥᑯᐸᔩᐦ ᐃᔅᑯᑖᒃ ᐹᐦᑫᑦ ᐊᓂᑌ ᔮᐸᑎᓯᔭᒡ᙮

*de bain, est-ce que ça va vraiment venir?* Le médecin lui dit que ça finirait par se remettre naturellement en place. Et ce fut le cas.

L'autre moitié du temps, elle pensait à d'autres choses. Une personne qu'elle aimait et qui avait été l'une de ses personnes préférées, s'était suicidée et Il y avait quelques éléments de cette situation qui n'avaient tout simplement pas de sens.

The other half the time, she was thinking about other things. Her cousin, who had been one of her favourite people, had committed suicide and there were a few things about that whole situation that just didn't make sense.

Elle pensait aussi à ses enfants. Son fils lui disait « Maman, tu me tues ! » quand le dîner était à nouveau composé d'aliments sains, avec beaucoup de légumes, mais il le mangeait quand même. Elle était une meilleure mère maintenant qu'elle était en meilleure santé. Elle aimait plus ses enfants et avait plus de patience pour leur façon d'être des enfants.

She thought about her kids too. "Mom, you're killin' me!" her son would say when dinner would again be something healthy with lots of vegetables, but he would eat it anyways. She was a better mom now that she was healthier. She liked her kids more and had more patience with the ways they were kids.

Parfois, elle pensait encore à son ancien chum. Il était parti, avait déménagé dans une autre communauté, pour être avec sa nouvelle famille. Jennifer était beaucoup plus mince qu'elle ne l'avait été. Les gens lui demandaient sans cesse si elle s'affamait. (Ce n'était pas le cas). Son médecin lui-même était tombé des nues lorsqu'elle était entrée dans son bureau.

Sometimes she still thought about her ex-boyfriend. He was gone, moved to another community to be with his new family. Jennifer was much smaller than she had once been. People kept asking her if she was starving herself. (She wasn't.) Even her doctor had had to pick up his jaw from the floor when she walked into his office. But she hadn't lost the

ᐊᓂᑖᐦ ᐅᒥᓯᓂᐦᐄᒑᐅᑭᒥᑯᔨᒡᐦ᙮ ᓂᒦᔮᔨᐤ ᐧᐋᐦᒋ ᒌᐦ ᐊᒋᐧᐃᐲᐦᐄᓰᑦ ᐅᐦᒋ ᐊᓂᔮᐦ ᑳ ᓂᑭᑎᑯᑦ ᑳ ᐱᐱᒋᐢᑭᓈᐱᔨᒡᐦ᙮ ᐧᐄᔨ ᐊᓂᔮᐦ ᒌᐦ ᐧᐄᐦ ᐧᐄᒋᐦᐄᓰ ᐊᑎᑎᐤ ᒑ ᒌᐦ ᒥᔪᒥᒋᐦᐅᑦ᙮ ᑖᐹ ᐊᑐᒡ ᐅᐦᒋ ᒋᐦ ᐃᐦᑐᑎᒻ ᐋᔥᒄ ᒌᐦ ᐃᐦᑖᔨᒡᐦ ᐊᓂᑎᐦ ᐋᐦ ᐃᐦᑖᒡ᙮

ᐹᔨᐧᑳᐤ ᒫᒃ ᐊᓂᔮ ᐋᐦ ᐱᐹᒧᐦᑖᑦ, ᐋᐦ ᒋᐢᒋᓰᑎᑎᐦᒃ ᒦᓰᐅᑭᒥᑯᔨᐤ ᑭᔮᐦ ᐊᓂᔮ ᒨᔮᒻ ᐋᐦ ᐅᔥᑳᔨᒡ ᐅᐱᒫᑎᓰᐧᐃᓐ, ᐋᑯᑎᐦ ᑳ ᒋᐢᒑᔨᐦᑎᐦᒃ ᐋᑳ ᒦᓐ ᑳᐤ ᒑ ᐧᐄᒑᐧᐋᑦ ᐊᓂᔮᐦ ᑳᐱᐱᒋᐢᑭᓈᐱᔨᒡᐦ᙮ ᐹᔨᐧᑳᐤ ᒌᐦ ᐧᐋᐱᒫᐤ ᐊᓂᑖᐦ ᐋᐦ ᒥᐦᒑᑎᓈᓂᐧᐃᐧᐃᔨᒡ ᑭᔮᐦ ᓈᔥᒡ ᐋᐦ ᒌᐦ ᑭᓂᐧᐋᐱᒥᒃᑯᑦ, ᐊᓂᔮ ᑭᔨᐧᐹ ᓈᔥᒡ ᐄᔨᐦᒡ ᔖᔥ ᐋᐦ ᐄᓯᓈᑯᓯᐧᐋᑦ᙮ ᐄᔑᓈᑯᓂᔨᒑ ᒫᒃ ᒑ ᓂᑭᑖᑦ ᐊᓂᔮᐦ ᑯᑎᒃᐦ ᐃᐢᐧᑳᐤᐦ ᑭᔮᐦ ᐊᓂᔮᐦ ᑯᑎᒃᐦ ᐅᑎᐧᐋᔑᔒᒻᐦ, ᐹᒋ ᓂᑎᐧᐋᐱᒥᑯᒑ ᑭᔮᐦ ᓈᔥᒡ ᓰᐦᒃ ᐄᑎᑯᒑ ᒦᓐ ᐋᐦ ᐧᐄᐦ ᐧᐄᒑᐅᑯᑦ, ᐊᑐᒡ ᐧᐄ ᓈᔥᑎᔨᒡ ᐃᔮᐱᑖᔨᒫᐤ᙮

ᓈᐦᐋᐤ ᒫᒃ ᒑᑳᑦ ᐋᐱᐦᑎᐤ ᐄᐢᑎᑎᐤ ᒉᓂᕙᕐ ᑳ ᒌᐦ ᐄᐢᑎᑎᒃ ᒫᐧᑳᒡ ᓈᑖᐦ ᒥᓅᓐᓛᓐ ᑳ ᐃᐦᑖᒡ ᓃᔕᐱᐳᓐᐦ ᐊᓂᑖᐦ ᐄᔑ ᐅᑖᐦᒡ᙮ ᓂᒧᐃ ᔖᔥ ᐋᐱᒋᐦᑖᐤ ᐊᓂᔮ ᓂᑐᐦᑯᔨᓐᐦ ᐋᐦ ᔖᑳᐅᐱᔨᓈᓂᐧᐃᐧᐃᔨᒡ ᑳ ᐋᐱᒋᐦᑖᑦ᙮ ᐋᔥᒄ ᓈᔥᒡ ᐧᐄᐦ ᒦᒋᐤ ᐋᐦ ᔒᐧᐋᔨᒡ ᒑᐧᑳᔨᐤ ᓂᔮᓂᑯᒎᓐᐦ, ᐊᓂᔮ ᒫᒃ ᐋ ᐃᐦᑎᐦᒡ, ᐊᐱᔒᔥ ᒫᒋᑦ ᐧᒑᑭᑕᑎᔨᐤ, ᓈᔥᒡ ᓈᐅᔥ ᐋᐦ ᒫᒫᑯᐦᑎᐦᒃ, ᑭᔮᐦ ᓂᒥ ᒦᓐ ᐊᑎᑎᐤ ᐱᐦᐧᑳᐦᑎᒻ ᑭᔮᐦ ᐧᐃᔮᐱᓂᐦᒃ ᐊᓂᔮ ᑳ ᐄᔥᑯᔥᑎᐦᒃ᙮

ᐊᓂᔮᐦ ᒫᒃ ᒑᐧᑳᔨᐤᐦ ᓈᔥᒡ ᐋᑳ ᐅᐦᒋ ᒌᐦ ᐴᓂᐦᑖᑦ, ᐋᔫᐧᐃᒄ ᒫᐅᒡ ᐧᑳᐢᐱᓈᔨᐦᑎᐦᒃ ᒦᓐ

ᓇᒧᐃ ᑮᐹ ᐅᐦᒋ ᐊᓂᔫ ᐅᐧᐁᐢᑲᒋᐱᓂᒻ ᑳ ᐧᐋᓴᑲᒥᑐᐧᐋᐱᔨᒡ ᐧᐁᐦᒌ ᐊᒎᐸᔨᑦ᙮ ᐧᐃᔭ ᒌᐧᐄ ᐧᐄᒋᐦᐄᓰᑦ ᒉᒌ ᒥᔫᐢᑲᐧᐄᑦ᙮ ᓇᒧᐃ ᓈᓂᑑ ᒋᐹᒌ ᐃᐦᑑ ᐁᐢᒄ ᒌ ᐧᐄᒉᐧᐋᑯᐸᓄ ᐊᓂᔫᐦ ᑳᒌ ᐧᐄᒉᐧᐋᑦ᙮

ᐯᔭᐧᑳᐤ ᐁ ᐱᒧᐦᑌᑦ ᒉᐧᑳᒡ, ᒌ ᒫᒥᑐᓀᔨᐦᑕᒻ ᐊᓂᔫ ᐁᑳ ᒌ ᒥᔫᐧᐁᐱᓇᐦᒃ ᒉᐧᑳᔫ ᒦᓰᐅᑲᒥᑯᐦᒡ ᐁ ᐃᑐᐦᑌᑦ ᑲᔦ ᐅᐱᒫᓯᒌᐧᐃᓐ ᐲᑐᔥ ᐁ ᐃᔑᓈᑯᓂᔨᒡ ᑖᓐ ᑳᐯᒋ ᐃᔑᓈᑯᓂᔨᒡ ᐊᓂᑌ ᐅᑖᐦᒡ᙮ ᑳ ᐃᑌᔨᐦᑕᐦᒃ ᐁᑳ ᒦᓐ ᑳᐤ ᒉ ᐅᐦᒋ ᐧᐄᒉᐧᐋᑦ ᑳ ᐧᐁᓴᑲᒥᑐᐧᐋᐱᔨᒡ᙮ ᒌ ᐧᐋᐸᒣᐤ ᐊᓂᑌ ᒉᐧᑳᔫ ᐁᒌ ᐃᐦᑑᑖᑲᓄᔨᒡ ᐁᒌ ᒥᐦᒉᑎᓈᓄᔨᒡ ᓈᔥᒡ ᐁᒌ ᑲᓇᐧᐋᐸᒥᑯᑦ ᐊᓂᔫ ᑮᐹ ᐴᑦ ᒥᐢᑕᐦᐄ ᐁᒌ ᐊᒎᐸᔨᑦ᙮ ᐋᑦ ᓇᑲᑖᔨᒡ ᐊᓂᔫ ᐧᐋᒋᒫᑦ ᑲᔦ ᐅᑕᐧᐋᔒᒻᐦ ᒦᓐ ᑳᐤ ᐧᐃ ᐯᒋ ᓈᔑᑦ ᓇᒧᐃ ᒦᓐ ᐧᐄᔥᑳᒡ ᓂᐹ ᐅᐦᒋ ᐧᐄᒉᐧᐋᐤ ᒌ ᐃᑌᔨᐦᑕᒻ᙮

ᐧᐃᔦᐢ ᐧᐋᐱᐦᑑ ᒌ ᐃᔥᐱᔥ ᐊᒎᐸᔫ ᑖᓐ ᑳ ᐃᔥᐱᒋᔥᑎᑦ ᐊᓂᑌ ᒪᓅᓐᓛᓐᑦ ᑳ ᐃᐢᐸᔨᐧᑖᐤ ᓃᔕ ᐱᐳᓐᐦ ᐊᓂᑌᐦ ᐃᔑ ᐅᑖᐦᒡ᙮ ᓇᒧᐃ ᐅᑎᓇᒻ ᓵᐢ ᐊᓂᔫ ᓂᑐᐦᑯᐃᓐᐦ ᐧᐁᑎᓇᐦᒃ ᐊᐧᐁᓐ ᐁ ᓰᐧᐋᑲᒥᐦᐧᒉᑦ᙮ ᐁᐢᒄ ᑮᐹ ᓂᔮᓂᑯᑌᐦᒡ ᐧᐃ ᓰᐅᒦᒋᓰ ᐅᔫ ᒫᒃ ᐁ ᐃᐢᐸᔨᑦ ᒥᒄ ᒋᔮᒻ ᐊᐱᔒᔥ ᐸᐦᐧᒉᑲᐦᑕᒻ ᐧᒑᑲᑕᑎᔫ, ᐧᐁᐃᐱᐢᒌᔥ ᒫᒫᑯᐦᑕᒻ ᐁᒄ ᒉ ᐊᐸᐦᑯᑌᐦᑕᐦᒃ᙮

ᐊᓂᔫᐦ ᒫᒃ ᒉᐧᑳᔫᐦ ᓵᐢ ᐁᒌ ᐴᓂᐦᑖᑦ ᐯᔭᒄ ᒉᐧᑳᔫ ᑯᔥᑕᒻ ᒦᓐ ᑳᐤ ᒉᒌ ᓰᐅᒦᒋᓰᑦ᙮ ᑯᔥᑕᒻ

Cependant, elle n'avait pas perdu le poids pour ce bon vieux Monsieur Les-yeux-bleus. Elle avait travaillé, pour elle-même, à se sentir bien dans son propre corps. Elle n'en aurait jamais été capable s'il avait été là.

weight for ol' Blue Eyes. She had done the work for herself to feel good in her own body. She would never have been able to do it if he had been around.

Lors d'une de ces promenades, alors qu'elle pensait à moitié à la salle de bain et à moitié à sa nouvelle vie, elle réalisa qu'elle n'accepterait pas que Monsieur Les-yeux-bleus revienne. Elle l'avait vu de l'autre côté de la foule lors d'un récent événement communautaire et il ne pouvait pas s'empêcher de la regarder, elle et ce dont elle avait l'air désormais. S'il quittait son autre famille et venait la supplier, jamais au grand jamais elle n'accepterait qu'il revienne.

On one of those walks, half thinking about the toilet and half thinking about her new life, she realized that she wouldn't take Blue Eyes back. She had seen him across the crowd at a recent community event and he couldn't stop staring at her, at how she looked now. If he left his other family and came to her and begged, she would never ever take him back.

Jennifer fait environ la moitié du poids qu'elle faisait lors de son voyage à Marineland il y a quelques années. Elle ne prend plus de médicaments pour le diabète désormais. Elle lutte toujours contre ses envies de sucre et, lorsqu'une envie devient incontrôlable, elle prend une ou deux bouchées d'une barre de chocolat, les mâche trèèèèèèèès lentement et jette le reste.

Jennifer is about half the weight she was on that trip to Marineland a couple of years ago. She doesn't take any diabetes medication now. She still fights sugar cravings, and, when a craving gets out of hand, she takes a bite or two of a chocolate bar, chews reeeaaaallllyyy slowly, and throws the rest away.

De toutes ses vieilles dépendances qui pourraient revenir, c'est la dépendance à

Of all her old addictions that might come back, she's most afraid of the junk food

ᓈᔥᒡ ᒫ ᐄᔑᑭᐦᒃ᙮ ᐋᐄᔫᐧᐃᒄ ᐊᓂᔮ ᓈᔥᒡ ᐧᑳᔅᐱᓈᔨᐦᑎᐦᒃ ᒥᔑᐤ ᐹᔨᐧᑳᐤ ᒦᒋᑖ ᐋᑳ ᒫ ᒌᐦ ᐴᓃᑦ ᑮᔮᐦ ᒦᓐ ᒫ ᐄᔥᐱᔑ ᑖᐦᒋᐳᑦ ᐊᓂᔮ ᑳ ᐄᔥᐱᔑ ᑖᐦᒋᐳᑦ ᐋᐦᐧᒫᔮᐦ ᐅᐦᒋ ᐴᓂᐦᑖᑦ ᑮᔮᐦ ᐅᐦᒋ ᐱᐹᒧᐦᑖᑦ᙮

ᒑᑳᑦ ᒨᔥ ᔔᔥ ᐧᐄᐦ ᒋᔅᒋᓰ = ᐧᐄᔨ ᑎᐹᔨᐦᑎᒻ ᐅᐱᒫᑎᓰᐧᐃᓐ᙮ ᑮᔮᐦ ᒋᔅᒑᔨᐦᑎᒻ ᓈᔥᒡ ᓈᓈᓂᒌᒡ ᐋᐦ ᐋᑎ ᒥᔪᐱᔨᑦ, ᐊᑎᑎᐤ ᓈᔥᒡ, ᓂᒧᐃ ᒦᓐ ᓂᐦᑖ ᒦᓐ ᓈᑖᐦ ᐧᐄᐦ ᐄᔑ ᐱᒫᑎᓰᐤ ᐊᓂᔮ ᑳ ᐄᔑ ᐱᒫᑎᓰᑦ ᓈᑖᐦ ᐄᔑ ᐅᑖᐦᒡ᙮

ᐧᐄᐦ ᐧᐋᐱᐦᑎᒻ ᐅᑖᐦ ᐄᔨᔨᐅᔅᒌᒡ ᐋᑳ ᓈᔥᒡ ᒫ ᐲᐦᑎᑖᐱᔨᔨᒡ ᓂᑎᐧᐄ ᐋᐦ ᐄᔑᓈᑯᓂᔨᒡ ᒫᐧᑳᔨᐤ ᐋᐦ ᒦᒋᓈᓂᐧᐃᐧᐃᔨᒡ, ᒥᓯᐧᐋ ᑭᔨᐧᐹ ᐊᐧᐋᔨᐤᐦ ᐋᐦ ᒋᔅᒋᓰᑎᑎᐧᐋᑦ᙮ ᒫ ᐧᐄᐦ ᓂᓯᑐᐦᑎᐦᒡ ᐊᐧᐋᓂᒌ ᐋᑳ ᒋᔥᒋᐧᐋ ᒦᒋᒥᐦᒡ ᐄᔑᓈᑯᓂᔨᒡ ᐅᔮ ᒫᐧᑳᔨᐤ᙮

ᒦᓐ ᒫᒃ ᑏᐧᐋᐦᒡ ᒫᐧᑳᔨᐤ ᒫᔅᒋᓰᑎᑎᐦᒃ, ᐋᔪᐧᐃᒄ ᐊᓂᔮ ᒫ ᐧᐄᐦ ᐴᓃᑦ ᐋᐦ ᐱᐦᐧᑖᑦ᙮ ᐋᔪᐧᐃᒄ ᒦᓐ ᒫᐧᑳᔨᐤ ᓈᔥᒡ ᒫ ᐋᔨᒥᓂᔨᒡ᙮ ᑮᔮᐦ ᐧᑳᐧᔔᓐ ᒦᓐ ᑯᑎᒋᔨᐤ ᒫᐧᑳᔨᐤ ᒋᑭ ᐧᐄᐦ ᐃᐦᑐᑎᒻ ᐊᓂᑎᐦ ᒫ ᒌᐦ ᐅᐦᒋ ᔔᔔᐧᐄᑦ᙮ ᐊᓂᔮ ᒫᐧᑳᔨᐤ ᒫ ᐧᐄᐦ ᒥᔥᑭᐧᐃᐦᐄᑯᑦ ᐅᔅᐱᑐᓂᐦᒡ ᑮᔮᐦ ᐊᑎᑎᐤ ᒫ ᒌᐦ ᒥᐧᔮᔅᑯᔨᐧᐋᑦ᙮ ᐄᐦᐄ, ᑖᐧᐹᐦ ᓈᑖᐦ ᐧᐋᔥᑭᒡ ᑖᐹ ᐅᐦᒋ ᐃᔨᓯᓈᑯᓯᐤ, ᒌᐦ ᒥᓯᒋᔅᑎᐤ ᑮᔮᐦ ᒥᓯᐧᐋ ᐊᐧᐋᔨᐤᐦ ᒌᐦ ᐧᐋᐱᒥᑰ᙮ ᒥᒄ ᒫᒃ ᒥᒄ ᒦᓐ ᐧᐄᐦ ᒥᐧᔮᔅᑯᔨᐧᐋᐤ, ᒦᓐ ᒫ ᒌᐦ ᒥᔪᓈᑯᓯᑦ, ᐋᑳ ᒦᓐ ᒫ ᑖᐦᒋᐳᑦ᙮

ᒦᒋᒥᔫ ᐁᑳ ᒥᔫᔅᑳᑫᔨᒡ ᑫᒌ ᒦᒋᑦ ᐧᐁᔥ ᒥᒋᐦᐱᓐ ᐯᔭᐧᑳᐤ ᒦᒋᑌ ᐁᐅᒄ ᒋᐦᒋᐧᐁ ᑫᐧᐄ ᐃᐦᑎᑦ ᑲᔦ ᑳᐤ ᒦᓐ ᑫ ᒥᓯᒋᔥᑎᑦ ᐁᑳ ᑯᐃᔅᑯ ᐃᔑ ᒦᒋᓯᑌ᙮

ᒋᔅᑫᔨᐦᑕᒻ ᑮᐹ ᓵᔅ ᒥᒍᓐ ᐧᐄᔭ ᑫᒌ ᐧᐃᔦᔨᐦᑕᒃ ᑖᓐ ᑫ ᐃᐦᑎᑦ ᐁᐧᐄ ᒥᔫᐱᒫᑎᓰᑦ᙮ ᓄᐧᐊᒡ ᒫᒃ ᐋᐦᒌᐅᐦ ᐃᐦᑑ ᐁᒄ, ᓈᔅᒡ ᑖᐧᐯ ᒥᔫᐸᔫ ᓇᒧᐃ ᒫᒃ ᒦᓐ ᑳᐤ ᐧᐄ ᓈᑕᒻ ᑖᓐ ᑳ ᐯᒋ ᐄᑖᑎᓰᒡ᙮

ᒋᐹ ᒥᔦᔨᐦᑕᒻ ᐁᑳ ᓈᔥᒡ ᐃᐦᑕᑯᓂᔨᒡ ᒦᒋᒥᔫ ᐁᑳ ᒥᔫᔅᑳᑫᔨᑦ ᐊᓂᑌ ᐄᓅ ᐊᔅᒌᐦᒡ᙮ ᒋᐹ ᒋᔅᑫᔨᐦᑕᒧᒡ ᐄᓅᒡ ᐁᑳ ᒥᒍᓐ ᒦᒋᒥᐦᒡ ᐃᑌᔨᐦᑖᑯᐦᒡ᙮

ᐁᒄ ᒦᓐ ᑯᑕᒋᔫ ᐧᐋᐦ ᐴᓂᐦᑖᑦ ᐁᐅᑯᔫ ᐁ ᐲᐦᐧᑖᑦ ᒋᔥᑌᒫᐤᐦ᙮ ᐁᐅᒄ ᒦᓐ ᓈᓂᑑ ᑫᐧᐄ ᐋᔨᒥᐦᐄᑯᑦ ᑫᒌ ᐴᓂᐦᐋᑦ᙮ ᑮᐹ ᐴᑦ ᑫᐧᐄ ᓈᓂᑐᐧᐁᔨᐦᑕᐦᒃ ᑖᓐ ᑫᒌ ᐃᐦᑎᑦ ᐃᔅᑯᑕᒃ ᒨᔑᐦᑖᑌ ᐁᐧᐄ ᐲᐦᐧᑖᑦ᙮ ᒋᐱᐦᒌ ᓴᓵᐅᐸᔨᐦᐆ ᑫᒌ ᒥᔅᑰᐦᐧᐋᑦ ᐧᐃᔫᓐᐦ, ᒧᔫᒻ ᐅᔅᐱᑐᓐᐦ ᑲᔦ ᐅᔔᑲᓐ᙮ ᒥᐦᑫᑐ ᐱᔨᓐᐦ ᐊᓂᑌ ᐯᒋ ᐅᑖᐦᒡ ᓈᔥᒡ ᒌ ᒪᐦᒋᔔᑲᓀᐤ ᒥᓯᐧᐁ ᒫᒃ ᐊᐧᐁᔫᐦ ᒌ ᐧᐋᐸᒥᑰ ᑖᓐ ᑳ ᐃᔅᐱᒋᔥᑎᑦ᙮ ᓂᐹ ᒥᔦᔨᐦᑌᓐ ᐧᐋᐸᐦᑖᑲᓅᐦᒡ ᐁ ᐃᔥᐱᔥ ᒥᔫᓈᑯᓯᔮᓐ ᐁᑳ ᒪᐦᒋᔔᑲᓀᔮᓐ ᒌ ᐃᑌᔨᐦᑕᒻ᙮ ᑫᒌ ᐧᐋᐸᐦᑖᑲᓅᐦᒡ ᐁ ᒥᔫᓈᑯᓯᔮᓐ, ᒥᔫᔅᑯᐧᐃᔮᓐ ᑲᔦ ᐁ ᒥᔅᑰᐱᒫᑎᓯᔮᓐ᙮

la malbouffe qu'elle craint le plus. Elle a surtout peur qu'un repas de malbouffe en entraîne un autre, puis un autre, et que tout ce poids et ces mauvaises habitudes concernant sa santé s'accumulent à nouveau.

addiction. Most afraid that one junk food meal will lead to another and then another and all that weight and unhealthiness will pile back on.

Mais la plupart du temps, elle sait – elle est responsable de sa vie. Et c'est tellement mieux désormais, tellement mieux, elle ne retournera *jamais* à ce mode de vie.

But most of the time she knows – she is in charge of her life. And it's so much better now, so much better, she ain't *never* goin' back to that way of living.

Elle aimerait que la malbouffe soit interdite pour tout le monde dans l'Eeyou Istchee. Les gens devraient être informés que ce n'est pas vraiment de la nourriture.

She'd like to see junk food restricted in Eeyou Istchee for everyone. Folks oughta know it isn't actually food.

Pour la prochaine étape, elle pense qu'elle pourrait cesser de fumer. Ce sera probablement très difficile aussi. Et peut-être qu'elle commencera à pratiquer d'autres types d'activités physiques. Comme ces exercices de musculation ou de résistance qui sculptent les bras et le cul. Il y a des années, elle avait un cul d'arbre de Noël et tout le monde le savait. Ce serait bien d'avoir un cul célèbre à nouveau. Un beau derrière de femme forte, en santé et que tout le monde envie.

Next up, she thinks, she might stop smoking. That'll probably be another tough one. And maybe she'll take up some other kinds of exercise. Like some of those weight or resistance exercises that sculpt your arms and ass. Years ago, she had a Christmas tree ass and everyone knew. It'd be good to have a famous ass again. A healthy, well-shaped, look-how-strong-I-am, famous ass.

Syllabic Chart ᐄᔨᔨᐅᔥᑖᐤ

Tableau de caractères syllabiques ᐄᓅᔥᑌᐤ

| | | | | | | | | |
|---|---|---|---|---|---|---|---|---|
| ᐁ e | | ᐃ i | ᐄ ii | ᐅ u | ᐆ uu | ᐊ a | ᐋ aa | |
| | ᐌ we | ᐎ wi | ᐐ wii | ᐒ wu | ᐔ wuu | ᐗ wa | | ᐙ waa |
| ᐯ pe | ᐺ pwe | ᐱ pi | ᐲ pii | ᐳ pu | ᐴ puu | ᐸ pa | ᐹ paa | ᑆ pwaa |
| ᑌ te | ᑗ twe | ᑎ ti | ᑏ tii | ᑐ tu | ᑑ tuu | ᑕ ta | ᑖ taa | ᑣ twaa |
| ᑫ ke | ᑴ kwe | ᑭ ki | ᑮ kii | ᑯ ku | ᑰ kuu | ᑲ ka | ᑳ kaa | ᒀ kwaa |
| ᒉ che | ᒒ chwe | ᒋ chi | ᒌ chii | ᒍ chu | ᒎ chuu | ᒐ cha | ᒑ chaa | ᒞ chwaa |
| ᒣ me | ᒬ mwe | ᒥ mi | ᒦ mii | ᒧ mu | ᒨ muu | ᒪ ma | ᒫ maa | ᒸ mwaa |
| ᓀ ne | ᓊ nwe | ᓂ ni | ᓃ nii | ᓄ nu | ᓅ nuu | ᓇ na | ᓈ naa | ᓎ nwaa |
| ᓓ le | ᓜ lwe | ᓕ li | ᓖ lii | ᓗ lu | ᓘ luu | ᓚ la | ᓛ laa | ᓨ lwaa |
| ᓭ se | ᓶ swe | ᓯ si | ᓰ sii | ᓱ su | ᓲ suu | ᓴ sa | ᓵ saa | ᔂ swaa |
| ᔐ she | ᔗ shwe | ᔑ shi | ᔒ shii | ᔓ shu | ᔔ shuu | ᔕ sha | ᔖ shaa | ᔣ shwaa |
| ᔦ ye | ᔯ ywe | ᔨ yi | ᔩ yii | ᔪ yu | ᔫ yuu | ᔭ ya | ᔮ yaa | ᔻ ywaa |
| ᕃ re | ᐧᕃ rwe | ᕆ ~~ri~~ | ᕇ ~~rii~~ | ᕈ ~~ru~~ | ᕉ ruu | ᕋ ra | ᕌ raa | ᕍ rwaa |
| ᕓ ve | ᐧᕓ vwe | ᕕ vi | ᕖ vii | ᕗ vu | ᕘ vuu | ᕙ va | ᕚ vaa | ᕛ vwaa |
| ᕞ the | ᐧᕞ thwe | ᕠ thi | ᕡ thii | ᕢ thu | ᕣ thuu | ᕤ tha | ᕥ thaa | ᕦ thwaa |

| | |
|---|---|
| ᐤ u | ᐦ h |
| ᑉ p | |
| ᑦ t | |
| ᒃ k | ᒄ kw |
| ᒡ ch | |
| ᒻ m | ᒧ mw |
| ᓐ n | |
| ᓪ l | |
| ᔅ s | |
| ᔥ sh | |
| ᔾ y | |
| ᕐ r | |
| ᕝ v/f/ph | |
| ᕪ th | |